Endometriosis
Healing from the Inside Out

Your Guide to Healing and Managing Endometriosis Through Gentle Natural Therapies

Pre-Launch Reviews

'This book could not have come into my life at a better time! Having been really poorly with complications due to endometriosis, I finally decided that going natural with products and trying to sort out my diet was non-negotiable. Like many though, I found it so overwhelming.

This book is methodical and well laid out such that it was easy to go back and find something particular to re-read. I found it to be very relatable to the real world, with achievable suggestions unlike advice I have read in other books which just seemed impossible.

The concepts are explained well but not patronisingly so! For me, if I understand the theory behind something then I am more likely to try it out, so I enjoyed reading the scientific stuff, all the while reinforcing the decision that it was the right way to go.

I loved the odd quotes that were thrown in- positive and motivating. I enjoyed reading the theories and quotes from other professionals and in particular the thoughts about the link between mind and body- something I had recently been starting to learn about. I liked the tone of the book because it felt personal and caring, I think due to the fact that the author has been through the horrendousness that is endometriosis herself!

Funnily enough, I had started looking at recipes for home made products just before I read this book- this I also found overwhelming. This book does contain some easy DIY recipes for non-toxic products but it also ensures you understand why using such ingredients is better for you, which I think is really important for encouraging you to make better choices.

The book gives suggestions on supplements which are good for endometriosis and a few of those supplements are repeated quite a bit under different headings. However, I can see why the author did this and actually I found it to be helpful to me because it explained how a particular supplement was beneficial for each area mentioned and drumming it in even further! I think this is helpful for making an informed decision on which ones you feel are best suited to you.

I have to note that I was pleased to see that the author understood surgery as sometimes being required, rather than trying to persuade the reader that it was always an unnecessary option. I also like that I felt reassured that this process takes some time. Makes me feel better about taking so long to get my head around it all and actually start doing something practical about it!

Overall, I found the content of this book to be like an 'endo 101' that I wish I could keep in my pocket and carry around with me! I will be re-reading it more than once in my quest to rid my life (mostly) of chemicals and I really hope that it's all worth it in the end.'

Jodie

'Thank you for writing this book. It has given me so much faith that I will be able to beat this disease. It has provided a real eye-opener of what may have caused my endo, which has always been distressing for me as no-one in my family has had it. The wealth of advice of all the things I can do to help myself is worth the price of the book alone, and the motivational messages and the stories of other women who have healed really gives credit to your message. Thank you'

Jilly, Arizona, US

'I was diagnosed with endometriosis over 5 years ago. I have had 2 laparoscopies to try and clear the endo, and tried various drug treatments, but the endo kept returning. After reading your book I decided not to continue with any more drug treatments - they always made me feel so awful. And what was the point, the endo was still there.

I changed my diet and started seeing improvement within 2 weeks, and after 6 weeks my endo pain was almost gone, just a bit of pain with my period. I also started seeing a Naturopath as I wanted to know I was doing thing correctly. I felt a bit worse at first as my Naturopath put me on a detox program to get rid of toxins in my system from all the drug treatments. But I am now seeing gradual improvements. My general health and stamina are improving as well as feeling so much better emotionally.'

Amada, Bristol, UK

'The honesty of the advice in your book have given me a real belief that I can get my own health back. I have started to make changes as suggested and already feel the benefits with a reduction in my pain and bloating. If I feel myself slipping back, I just have to read the success stories in the book and I feel more optimistic and ready to fight back. Thank you for your honesty, for sharing your own story of dealing with endo, and for writing this book which I feel has been a life saver for me.'

Claire, Cambridge, UK

'I have had endo for about 4 years now and have read many books on the subject. Some were quite good (good for reference purposes), some have been average, and others I felt were useless - especially those too full of medical jargon. Your book is the first one I have read, which in my opinion is accurate, practical, very supportive, and not too biased - or if it was in places, at least it was honest!!

I would recommend this book to all women with endometriosis because it is comprehensive in its content, very well researched and written, and most importantly it has given me hope and reassurance that healing can happen, and I now have the inspiration to fight this disease using my own resources. Many, many thanks.'

Dinah, Florida, US

'I have read many books on the subject of endo and have suffered from this for 10 years! mostly undiagnosed! This book is by far the best in terms of research and facts. Carolyn suffered from endo herself and is well versed in the devastating life changing effects it can have. I have changed my diet and my outlook thanks to her and have noticed a huge difference in my symptoms! Please read this if you have endo! it will give you hope and help you to feel less alone with this horrible disease!'

Angela, USA

'Having read a number of books that deal with natural treatments for endometriosis, this is by far the best one I have read. Not only is it very comprehensive in all aspects of natural treatments and self-help ideas for endometriosis, it is also VERY inspirational. The authors own story of defeating endometriosis in the first section has given me lots of hope that I can also get on top of this disease.

The book is written in a very supportive way and is packed full of tips and ideas that other books don't cover, like dealing with finances, a detailed look at causes of fatigue, how to stay motivated, and also covers fascinating chapters on the immune system and healing.

This book has been clearly researched including extensive references to reliable sources of information, and links subjects together so that you get a good overview and understanding of this disease and how natural treatments can and do really help. This book has given me the inspiration to work on my own health. An excellent book all round and I am very glad I found it and I highly recommend it to any woman who has endometriosis.'

Heather, Nottingham, UK

'I'm just in love with this book. Such an eye opener. Knowing that there really is hope to treat this disease naturally is so comforting and the author being so candid about her own journey and life is wonderfully refreshing and I know she understands. I started my journey 2 days before reading this book. I find it hard sticking with healthy plans because of the constant fatigue and outside influences but this book has made my mind over and I am going to do some serious life changes.

I love the part how our cells are listening to us so I am really going to try and be mentally positive. I really enjoyed the testimonials throughout the book of how different remedies helped them.

I knew about benefits of serrapeptase for the plaque in the arteries but didn't know it could help with endo so I will try that. It really sounds promising and logical to me now.

Thank you so much for giving me the opportunity to read this book. I have to read it again now to make notes. There are a lot of gems I need to write down. Everything I need to know is in this book which means no painstaking research over countless websites. You can focus on what you want to try straight away. I can read just this book and start my journey.'

Ruth, USA

We can heal ourselves beautifully and the body does a brilliant job if it is given the chance. To quote Deepak Chopra from his book '*Quantum Healing*':

> '.......... *we already know that the living body is the best pharmacy ever devised. It produces diuretics, painkillers, tranquillisers, sleeping pills, antibiotics, and indeed everything that is manufactured by the drug companies, but it makes them much, much, better. The dosage is always right and given on time; side effects are minimal or non-existent; and the directions for using the drug are included in the drug itself, as part of its built-in intelligence.*'

Every five days our whole intestinal lining is renewed. You make a new liver every 6 weeks. A new skin once a month. Every six months we have a new bloodstream. A complete new set of bones within 2 years. Even our brain cells are replaced. The DNA that holds memories of millions of years of evolution, even that is replaced every six weeks.

Now let's see if we can kick start your body to repair and renew itself!

ENDOMETRIOSIS
HEALING FROM THE INSIDE OUT

Your Guide to Healing and Managing Endometriosis
Through Gentle Natural Therapies

By

Carolyn Levett NT, BA

Disclaimer: The material in this book is intended as an educational tool to offer information about your options available for natural remedies and treatments to help the symptoms of endometriosis. The advice in this book is intended solely for informational and educational purposes only and not as medical advice. Please consult a medical professional if you have questions about your health.

Dedication

This book is dedicated to all the brave women and girls in the world who battle with endometriosis every day. Their stories of pain, suffering and distress led to the writing of this book – to give others hope and encouragement that they too could improve their health and start to reduce the impact this disease has on their life.

Contents

Foreword

This book is for women who are looking for hope and inspiration so they can start to achieve relief from the distressing disease of endometriosis and start to heal their body. I hope you find the advice here will provide an antidote against all the negative information you may have heard or read about your long-term prospects of dealing with this disease.

Time and time again you have been told that endometriosis is 'not curable'

What is a 'cure' anyway? The word 'cure' is very loaded with expectations and assumptions. Would you be happier if we used the word healing, remission, or recovery? Whichever word you prefer - you do have the ability to improve your health and start to eliminate your symptoms. Myself and many other women have had success by using natural therapies and self-help strategies to help regain our health.

You have an in-built natural support mechanism on your side
– your immune system

This book is not written by another medical professional who has their own 'view' on natural remedies for this disease. It is not another book about 'coping strategies.' This book is written by someone who had the disease, overcame the disease, and now aims to pass on much needed positive advice and support to other women.

When I was diagnosed, I was told by my gynaecologist that I had one of the worst cases of endometriosis she had seen and that I was in a complete mess internally. Her prognosis was not good at all. Her suggested method of treatment was just as bad. I reeled with shock at first, but I soon gathered my energies, learnt of my treatment options, collected information about the disease and gradually found my own path towards the goal of healing myself. It was not a quick fix; repairing and healing the body takes time, patience, commitment and faith.

Knowing there is so much negative information about endometriosis, my aim has been to redress this imbalance and help to motivate others of the notion that using natural therapies has much to offer. This has been achieved through my website, and this book is a natural progression of that process.

It saddens me to keep reading 'There is no cure for endometriosis'. That puts women on the back foot before they even start. It instils the mis-belief that you cannot regain your health.

Yes, you can – you can start to heal your body, and given enough support, by including natural therapies, supporting your body through nutrition, ensuring you remove toxins, combined with getting your immune system working on all four cylinders – you have a very good chance.

Lastly, you will find a number of books focussing on natural treatment concepts to manage endometriosis, each with their own viewpoint or emphasis. It can be difficult to write a book that suits everyone as we obviously have different opinions and experiences. The advice here has been written with integrity and honesty, so as not to misguide anyone or give false hope. This is not a medical manual, or a 'quick-fix' guide.

This is a resource providing sign-posts to many different natural remedies and self-help measures you can use to support your health. I just hope you can gain enough inspiration and advice in the pages here to give you a head-start on your own journey to managing this disease more naturally.

About the Author

Endometriosis is an all-encompassing disease and affects every aspect of a woman's life, which is something I fully understands. This is why I feel personally qualified to be able to offer guidance and support to those seeking advice and reassurance when dealing with this disease.

I am a qualified Integrative Health Coach having gained qualifications in Nutritional therapy, Naturopathy, Aromatherapy and Counselling. These skills have provided me with the knowledge to successfully help other women to manage their endometriosis naturally and recover their health.

I have been offering advice and support through my website at endo-resolved.com for over 10 years, which has provided guidance and encouragement for thousands of women wishing to go the natural route to support their health.

A number of my articles have appeared in various sources including Everyday Health, Endometriosis News, Livestrong, Healthy Women and Hormones Matter. Additionally, I am the author of the endometriosis cookbook 'Recipes & Diet Advice for Endometriosis' which has helped many get on track with an anti-inflammatory diet to help reduce their symptoms.

A bit of background from the author

You need to note that I am not a medical expert when it comes to endometriosis. The advice and content of this book is based on my own experience, as well as my research, backed up by my training in natural therapies.

The guidance in this book describes a multi-faceted approach to healing and recovering your health. This was the approach that worked for me and allowed me to get my life back on track, despite being diagnosed with severe endometriosis.

Please be aware that the advice here is not to be seen as a substitute for professional medical advice and you should always consult your physician when it comes to your health.

You may have other health problems additional to endometriosis, and you need to ensure you maintain medical supervision to monitor your health.

For legal purposes I am unable to make any claims to the efficacy and principles contained within this book. I have only been able report what has worked for me plus the addition of first-hand feedback from others who have had success. Everyone is individual and you need to take responsibility for your own health and ensure you maintain medical guidance from your doctor.

To conclude, I am passionate about encouraging women with endometriosis to help them heal their bodies and overcome this disease without having to rely on toxic drugs and surgeries, which can often cause further damage.

I hope that by sharing my knowledge combined with my own experience, you can start your own journey towards improving your health and begin to live a better and healthier life.

with healing thoughts,

Carolyn Levett Dip NT, BA

BEFORE WE GO ON ...

Breathe deep

Relax your jaw

Drop your shoulders

Relax your fists

And breathe deep again

Hopefully your tension should now
be released

A Brief Account Of My Story

When I was diagnosed with endometriosis, it was 2 weeks before Christmas and after I recovered from my surgery and was preparing to go home, I was told by the nurse to come back after the holidays to have 'a chat' with my gynaecologist to discuss the outcome of my surgery.

I went home feeling some sense of apprehension, but relieved the surgery was over and done. I anticipated my diagnosis to be something manageable and easy to treat ..... little did I know!

My symptoms were not severe – I had just been feeling very 'off' for a long time, weak, tired and very run-down. My periods were more painful than they should be and tended to be a lot heavier than normal which was the main symptom that alerted me that something was wrong. I also had some nasty gut issues which included distressing abdominal bloating and had many bad reactions to certain foods with pain and discomfort.

On returning to the hospital just after Christmas I was informed I had very severe endometriosis and my abdominal cavity was full of cysts and adhesions and if I was not considering having children then I should contemplate having a hysterectomy.

BAM – I was not expecting that!!! Merry Christmas Carolyn

My gynaecologist said she felt the best course of action was to put me on drug therapy to put my periods on hold to try and get the disease to calm down, and then she could operate again and try to remove the disease. I was advised to think things over and go back in two weeks.

This time I went home, and to say I felt numb and shocked is an understatement.

It took me a few days to get to grips with my thoughts and the roller-coaster of my emotions. I did some quick research into the drug treatment being offered and after learning of the side effects, decided not to go back to my gynaecologist – ever! Over the following months I researched in earnest, to learn more about a disease I had never heard of till now. I contacted my local endometriosis group for advice and information and learned all I could about this disease.

I was fortunate that many of my friends, like myself, were interested in natural therapies, and one friend was in contact with a qualified homeopath and advised I contacted her. I had already tried a few basic remedies like supplements and aromatherapy, but I knew I needed some form of natural therapy that could work on a deep level of healing. I also knew I needed help going through this and not to be left struggling on my own.

During the first meeting I had with Julia, the homeopath, I knew I was in the right place. I had a two-hour consultation with her and we discussed many details of my health, my medical history, my likes and dislikes and many more questions that allowed her to get a good insight into me as a person both physically and mentally.

This was the start of my two-year healing journey going the natural route. At the same time, I started to research issues that could worsen endometriosis and learnt about diet and nutrition and the connection with disease and inflammation. I was already eating a mostly vegetarian diet with the occasional fish and chicken dish.

I was however eating a lot of dairy and had a particular weakness for cheese. I used to love mac and cheese as well as cauliflower cheese. In fact, I used to put grated cheese on top of many savoury dishes (yeiks!). Then after learning how dairy could cause inflammation, I felt it would be wise to help my health if I cut right back on my dairy consumption. I was very relieved to find that this helped considerably to reduce the pain and bloating I used to suffer.

I continued to find out more about diet and learnt about gluten being a possible cause of many health issues and possibly causing inflammation in the body. So, I decided to cut out gluten from my diet, and to my relief found this improved my fatigue and brain fog immensely along with helping to reduce my gut distress even further.

After starting treatments with my homeopath, I had an initial improvement, but then I started to feel really weak and very, very fatigued. I asked Julia why things were going in this direction and she explained that I was going through a healing stage where symptoms can become worse as the body is working on a deep level of healing.

This feeling continued for a few months, and then gradually my energy and health started to improve. This was a great relief and instilled confidence that I was heading in the right direction with my health.

I continued in earnest learning about endometriosis, natural therapies, nutrition, and healing, as well as continuing my homeopathic treatment over the following year. My health steadily and gradually improved, with the improvement in my energy and reduction in pain being major bench-marks as to how my health was gradually recovering. I was very prudent to try and keep my stress levels down, because whenever I did have a stressful episode my symptoms would become noticeably worse. I regularly used meditation, calming techniques and aromatherapy to help calm my system.

Around the two-year mark after my initial diagnosis my health was better than it had been in a long time. I had energy, little to no pain, my cycle was easy to manage with very little pain and my life was finally getting back on track.

However, I felt something was amiss. I could not put my finger on it. I felt fit and healthy but something was *off*. I tried to ignore this strange inner feeling, but it would not go away. I talked to my GP, who was fortunately on-board with me using natural therapies to manage my endometriosis (a rare situation). I asked if I could have a follow-up laparoscopy to 'see what was happening', and he said OK, and got me booked in for a second laparoscopy.

My follow-up laparoscopy was scheduled a few months later and I was lucky to have a surgeon with up to date training. I had my surgery as scheduled and when the surgeon came round the hospital ward to see me, he said I had one cyst on my ovary which he removed, but he said all the other cysts, adhesions and signs of endometriosis had literally dried up and there were no signs of any active endometriosis.

I recovered from that surgery very quickly, probably due to my immune system working at full force. And that was the last of any treatment I had for endometriosis – *and it never returned.*

My health continued in good shape and I went back to living my life. I did not need to have any further homeopathic treatments, but I continued with my new diet regime as I felt the benefits were worth the health improvements it provided.

The fact that my second laparoscopy provided proof that my endometriosis had cleared up, was evidence enough to want to provide motivation and support to other women who were going through this ordeal.

Healing can happen – and you have many options to help reduce your symptoms, increase your energy and get your health back on track.

To sum up - the combination of different strategies that helped me to recover my health

These included:

- Support from homeopathy which aided in supporting my immune system, helped me to manage the emotional impact and assisted in addressing imbalances in my body
- Changing my diet to ensure I was not eating foods that could trigger inflammation and pain, and eating foods that would support my system
- Supporting my body with specific supplements
- Working on reducing stress and prioritizing my health with lots of self-care

A little insight into my personal circumstances at the time...

You may be wondering what my particular circumstances were when I had endometriosis - a question I would ask too. Knowing some of my individual circumstances helps to put my story into context and helps to understand the resources (or lack of) I had at the time.

To explain very briefly - my own circumstances were not eased by financial comfort or privilege or being in a secure position to help me manage this disease.

I had various financial and stressful issues to deal with, including bailiffs coming to my house as I could not afford to pay my local taxes. I had to ration my trips to see my homeopath because of limited finances and I did have to stop working for a while (but I was glad to leave my job, which I ended up hating after five changes in job description and a new, uncaring manager, which really affected me emotionally).

I was single and living on my own and had no help on the home front apart from emotional support from friends. My living accommodation was far from ideal at the time needing repairs and very hard to heat in the winter. Not a great combination of factors to help really. I had to be self-reliant and sometimes had to live on my wits. When I had enough energy, I had to take on menial cleaning jobs to help me get through financially.

I had issues from my past to deal with from childhood like abandonment and abuse, and a family not understanding what I was going through with endometriosis and therefore not providing any support. I know that many of you have had to deal with various distressing problems in life, and now being diagnosed with this disease leaves you feeling overwhelmed, helpless, angry, bitter, resentful – just to name a few emotions.

Endometriosis really is a beast and it takes so much from you – which is why you need to dig deep to find the energy and resources to take on this disease. I hope some of the tools I offer here will provide the support and motivation you need to help you get your health back on track.

That was tough to write, and harder to include here—but I felt it
may help add to the conviction of my advice

About the advice here....

Like I said in the introduction, this is a guide of how to start using natural therapies and lifestyle changes to help you control your endometriosis and start to heal. This does not replace any medical advice and you should always seek guidance from your doctor if you are aiming to try any new health or medical regime.

We are all different and the way our bodies react to any remedies or treatment will be different. There is no 'one size fits all' when trying to fix the body. You need to do your research, and ensure there are no contra-indications regarding any treatment or drugs you are using at the moment.

This guide is not offered as a cure, but with patience and commitment, you will hopefully reap the benefits by going down a more natural route to help you manage this disease.

Success stories from others have been woven through the book to provide you with more confidence and maybe help you decide which remedies you wish to try for yourself.

You have already read my story of how I was able to achieve total healing, and like I said earlier, others have been able to reduce their symptoms with some gaining total remission — hang on to that thought!

'Don't get discouraged: it is often the last key in the bunch that opens the lock'

What Is Endometriosis?

The aim of this book is not about going into lengthy details about endometriosis, diagnosis methods, treatment options and so on, as there are many other books and online resources covering those topics. The focus here is about providing a resource about natural ways to manage this disease. However, I felt this overview would help to provide an introduction to your journey.

So, what is endometriosis ......

According to Lara Briden, the author of the 'Period Repair Manual', she feels that endometriosis is a whole-body inflammatory immune disease, and that part of the successful treatment plan needs to address imbalances of the immune system. I also share a similar viewpoint, especially for the need to treat the whole body, and not just the 'diseased parts.'

Physically what happens .....

Endometriosis is a biological malfunction which focuses on the reproductive organs and the pelvic region of a woman's body.

This disease will start quietly, insidiously and unnoticed. Then gradually, symptoms of painful periods, pain at other times of the month, and a general feeling of being run-down, will start to develop.

In women with endometriosis, the natural bodily processes of the reproductive system go seriously wrong. The disease is linked to and affected by the menstrual cycle and also affected by the immune system.

It is estrogen in the body, as well as external sources of estrogen that feeds the disease, and once it has taken hold it will encourage further growth of the disease with the development of cysts. These cysts can then grow and start to cause adhesions in the pelvic cavity.

Endometriosis - the enigmatic disease of the modern age!

- Endometriosis is one of the most far-reaching, devastating and misunderstood diseases in the world today.
- It is estimated that there are over 176 million women and girls who suffer from the disease world-wide. No doubt there are many more due to the number of women who have not been diagnosed.
- This number is growing all the time. It is more common than breast cancer and many other diseases that are well known. Despite the huge numbers of women who suffer from this disease, few people have actually heard of it, but this is gradually changing, though very slowly.

Becoming more common ...

This disease is becoming more and more common. This could be for a variety of reasons:

The methods of detecting and diagnosing endometriosis are improving all the time, so statistics reflect this as growing numbers of cases are detected.

The seriousness of the disease is gradually gaining momentum and more people are finally beginning to hear about it. This may be through television programs, magazine articles, the internet, or talking to friends.

1. So, there is an ever-increasing public awareness. This public awareness helps to alert women who have concerns about their health, especially regarding pelvic and menstrual pain, and more women are able to determine whether they have endometriosis.
2. More women are taking their pelvic pain and period pain seriously, rather than thinking of it as normal, consequently they are pursuing answers from the medical profession.
3. Finally, the numbers of women who have the disease appears to be increasing, especially in the last 30 years or so. It also appears to be more common in industrial countries, where pollution is higher.

How the disease starts

Physically, what happens is that tiny, and sometimes microscopic particles that are similar to the lining of the womb, are found in other parts of the body but mainly in the pelvic cavity. These particles behave in the same manner as the lining of the womb. The lining of the womb is called the endometrium, which is where this disease gets its name.

The natural process of the endometrium is to react with hormones produced in the body and each month the endometrium builds up with blood cells and other chemicals to prepare for pregnancy. When pregnancy does not occur then the endometrium sheds this blood and women have a period.

A similar reaction takes place in the stray cells that have found their way into the pelvic cavity. Each month they react to hormones, and break down and bleed, but the blood and tissue shed from these endometrial growths has no way of leaving the body. This results in internal bleeding, breakdown of the blood and tissue from these sites and leads to inflammation.

This process continues for months, or even years before symptoms of serious pain begins to develop. Many women start to suspect something is wrong because the amount of pain they feel with their periods. It will become worse as the months go by. It is then that women start to investigate and question the state of their health.

For other women the disease may not throw up any noticeable symptoms, but they may be having problems with their fertility and are not successful in conceiving. It is then that they seek medical advice which could lead to having a laparoscopy. It is during this procedure that the disease may be found.

As time goes by, this disease will progress and start to do more damage in the pelvic cavity. Eventually it can lead to scar tissue formation, adhesions, bowel problems, as well as a gradual decline in general health.

The disease in context

Essentially, it appears that the body, and its natural healing processes are defective. It can strike women at any time of their reproductive life but we are seeing more and more cases of young girls who have the disease.

Recent studies are beginning to indicate that women with the disease are at greater risk of other health problems, but this could be an indicator that women with this disease are actually suffering from a break-down in the immune system. This situation seems to 'ring true' as many women who have the disease seem to suffer from a myriad of other health problems.

It is affecting millions of women around the world today. It not only affects her health, it also affects quality of life, possibilities of having children, income earning potential, emotional well-being, relationships, sex life, economics issues where women live in a country where they have to pay for treatment, and social life; in essence it affects the entire lives of women.

Little progress has been made in the medical field in relation to obtaining a timely diagnosis or successful treatment - despite its significance as an increasing world-wide health problem. Most of the treatment available today revolves around the management of pain, drug intervention of the reproductive cycle and surgery to cut out the diseased tissue and removal of adhesions that can occur in the abdomen.

There is currently no mainstream medical procedure or treatment that is guaranteed to remove the disease for good. In many cases, after chemical or surgical intervention, there may be a short period of relief, but often the disease returns. This leads to women have recurring surgeries – with an added issue of additional scarring caused by surgery, and surgery always carries risks.

These are the hard facts that surround this disease today. Many women suffer for years and years. They may have one surgical procedure after another. They may spend thousands of dollars on treatment, especially if their health insurance does not cover it. They may travel miles in pursuit of sympathetic and informed medical treatment.

But there are some glimmers of hope beginning to appear. Many women today are beginning to take care of their own health with regard to dealing with this disease. Also, there are more doctors who are beginning to specialise in the disease, and new surgical techniques are being developed and these are helping to improve success rates with treatment.

Hope and self help

Hope and courage for many women is gained through sharing information and advice, and this helps them to stop feeling so alone.

Many self-help ideas and tips are being exchanged between sufferers through forums and support groups. This often includes feedback on the best endometriosis surgeons, and advice and feedback about natural treatments, supplements, diet changes and simple life-style changes that have helped. All these tips and helpful suggestions add up and can give hope to women that there are always options.

The foundations for good health: Good nutrition, good sleep, move your body, reduce your exposure to toxins and stress management

Theories Of The Cause

Here is a brief overview of some of the various theories as to the cause of this disease, which helps to put this disease into context.

There are many theories to the cause of endometriosis, but it seems no one really knows what triggers this disease. Let's have a look at some of the speculated theories.

Retrograde menstruation – this has now been totally dismissed

The retrograde menstruation theory - is the movement of menstrual flow, including sloughed endometrial tissue, back through the fallopian tubes into the peritoneal cavity during menstruation.

Retrograde menstruation has been documented in a variety of surgical studies, and it is estimated to occur in 90% of all menstruating women. So, if retrograde menstrual blood is being blamed as the cause of endometriosis, *then most women on the planet should have it.*

For most women, menstrual tissue debris that enters the peritoneal cavity is destroyed before the tissue can implant in the peritoneal cavity. <u>It is destroyed by the immune system</u>. If retrograde menstruation is so common, with almost all women experiencing it to some degree with each cycle, why do only 10% to 15% of women develop endometriosis?

The other problem with the theory of retrograde menstruation is that endometriosis has been found in other parts of the body, including the lungs, brain, limbs and even the eyes. This theory also does not account for the cases of endometriosis found in men who have been taking estrogen as part of treatment for prostate cancer.

Immune system response

Immune system response - In women without endometriosis, ectopic implants of endometrial tissue are destroyed by a variety of immune and inflammatory reactions. These include activation of the cell-mediated immune system, including an increase in the production and activation of cytotoxic T cells that respond to foreign invaders, and the stimulation of natural killer cells. Those with endometriosis have lower T cells to fight this invasion.

Inflammatory response

Inflammatory response - The damage, infertility and pain produced by endometriosis may be due to an over-active response by the immune system to the early presence of endometrial implants. The body, perceiving the implants as hostile, launches an attack. Levels of large white blood cells (called macrophages) are elevated in endometriosis. Macrophages produce very potent factors, which include cytokines (particularly those known as interleukins) and prostaglandins. Such factors are known to produce inflammation and damage in tissues and cells.

Growth factors

Growth factors - Vascular endothelial growth factor (VEGF) is secreted by endometrial cells. Under normal circumstances, VEGF is secreted within the uterus. When oxygen levels drop following menstruation and blood loss, VEGF levels rise and promote the growth of new blood vessels. This process is important for repairing the uterus following menstruation.

When endometrial cells land outside the uterus, however, investigators theorise that this same process occurs with unfortunate results. The cells secrete VEGF when they are deprived of blood and oxygen, which in turn stimulates blood vessel growth. In this case, however, blood vessel growth serves to promote implantation outside the womb.

Thyroid link

Thyroid Link - Some researchers believe that some women with endometriosis may be suffering from thyroid dysfunction. In one survey of the thyroid function and endocrine levels (hormones secreted from the glands of the pituitary) of 120 women with endometriosis, it was found that although their routine thyroid tests were normal, the incidence of thyroid auto-antibodies was 20% higher than the reported percentage in other women.

In some cases, the levels of thyroid auto-antibodies were consistent with a definite thyroid auto-immune disease. Some of these women were treated with low-dose thyroxin and the women's health improved considerably. (*More on this further*)

Liver disorders

Liver Disorder - Some people believe that liver disorders are the key in predisposing a woman to this disease. The liver is a filter of sorts. It detoxifies our body, protecting us from the harmful effects of chemicals, elements in food, environmental toxins, and even natural products of our metabolism. The liver also regulates and removes estrogen from the body through a series of processes.

Anything that impairs liver function or ties up the detoxifying function will result in excess estrogen levels. This can happen whether it has a physical basis as in liver disease, or an external cause as with exposure to environmental toxins, drugs, or dietary substances. Estrogen is produced not only internally but also produced in reaction to chemicals and other substances in our food. When it is not broken down adequately, higher levels of estrogen build up.

Hereditary Cause

Preliminary study results indicate that patients with relatives who have endometriosis may be genetically predisposed to develop it themselves. This theory was suggested as early as 1943. There is research currently underway on this theory.

I do feel that this avenue of thought has a stronger case regarding a predisposition for the disease, and not that the disease is passed on from one generation to the next. There will be many, many women who are the only ones in their family to develop this disease. There was no history of endometriosis in my own family.

Estrogen dominance

This is a very popular theory for the progression of endometriosis. Many women, not just those who have endometriosis, are estrogen dominant today. This is caused by the excess estrogen in the environment which is found in the food chain and by xeno-estrogens found in chemicals.

Another strong factor for the increase of estrogen in the environment is through the increased use of the birth control pill (BCP). When women are on the BCP they are ingesting hormones into their system including estrogen. Not all these hormones stay in the body and are excreted in urine.

This then goes into the water treatment systems and in turn is then re-distributed back into the domestic water system. This includes drinking water, and even though it is purified, there will still be trace amounts of estrogen that are unfiltered.

It is not possible to remove all chemicals and toxins during the purification process. This excess of estrogen in the environment is thought to encourage the development of endometriosis.

Endometriosis & Dioxins

There have been extensive studies looking at the link between endometriosis and environmental pollution and chemicals in the environment. The use of chemicals has increased dramatically in the past few decades.

These chemicals then enter the food chain as well as the general environment. It is now being speculated that this increase in chemicals could be one factor that is causing endometriosis, or at least increasing the numbers of women and girls who are now developing the disease.

Our bodies are now surrounded by many toxic chemicals every day. These come from the air we breathe, the water we drink, from our food chain, from the harsh chemical-based toiletries we use and the many house-hold cleaners we use in our homes.

Many of these chemicals can mimic the action of estrogen when they are absorbed by the body. One group of chemicals that has caused much concern is Dioxin. Dioxin is classed in the group of chemicals known as a Persistent Organic Pollutant (POP) - they are toxic, persistent (do not break down in the environment) and are bio-accumulative (stored in the body).

'Dairy is the second largest contribution of dioxin in our diet. Researchers speculate that women who don't have endometriosis have immune cells in the peritoneal cavity that destroy endometrial cells or discourage their growth. The presence of dioxins and other chemicals may change how this immune response functions, which can result in the unregulated growth of endometrial cells. Other research has shown that dioxins and other pollutants can disrupt how hormones work, which could contribute to endometriosis.'

From Dr Cook – Endometriosis specialist

What are dioxins?

Dioxins are a group of chemical compounds arising either naturally or more often as a by-product of industrial activities. Dioxins are formed in the manufacture of herbicides and pesticides, and also in combustion processes such as commercial or municipal waste incineration, burning of chlorine-containing substances and fuels such as wood, coal, diesel or oil, and even household fires.

Dioxins may be transported over considerable distances when dispersed into the air, which is the main pathway into the environment and ultimately the food chain. Dispersal in water is initially more local i.e., settlement in sediments from where they can eventually enter the food chain.

The main concern with dioxins is that they accumulate in fatty tissue in the body and are very persistent (i.e., they do not breakdown very easily). Exposure to very low levels of dioxins (parts per trillion) over long periods can contribute to reproductive and developmental problems and damage the immune system. In other words, it only takes low levels over time to cause disruption to health.

Foods high in animal fat, such as milk, meat, fish and eggs are the main source of dioxins for humans which are stored in fatty tissues and are neither metabolised nor excreted – in other words they stay in the body.

Another source of dioxins

As well as being found in the food chain, dioxins are also found in tampons. Studies have found trace amounts of dioxins in a number of tampon products and the pathologist Dr P Tierno of NYU believes that the cumulative long-term effect of using tampons can cause negative health effects.

To reduce exposure to dioxins

I do not think we can totally protect ourselves to exposure from dioxins, especially as they can spread as air-borne particles, and scientists have even found dioxins in the Antarctic. However, there are certain measures you can take to help protect yourself.

The most obvious way to reduce your exposure to dioxins is by reducing your consumption of animal products, especially high fat animal foods like dairy and fatty meat. Also, you need to change to safer natural period products, which is a topic we go into more detail further on.

Another way to help protect yourself from dioxins is drinking green tea, as research has found that green tea can help the body to eliminate dioxins from the body.

Today, more than 95% of all chronic disease is caused by food choice, toxic food ingredients, nutritional deficiencies and lack of physical exercise. Mike Adams

Diseases Of The Immune System

I strongly believe that endometriosis has its roots in a compromised immune system, especially as so many women with endometriosis also suffer from other diseases, many of which tend to be auto-immune diseases.

Auto-Immune Disease

The term "auto-immune disease" refers to a varied group of more than 80 serious, chronic illnesses that involve almost every human organ system. It includes diseases of the nervous, gastrointestinal, and endocrine systems as well as skin and other connective tissues, eyes, blood, and blood vessels. In all of these diseases, the underlying problem is similar- the body's immune system becomes misdirected, attacking the very organs it was designed to protect.

Many individual auto-immune diseases are rare, as there are many different types of auto-immune diseases. As a group, however, they afflict millions of people. Most auto-immune diseases affect women more often than men, particularly affecting women of working age and during their childbearing years.

Auto-Immune Reactions

Auto-immune reactions can be triggered in several ways:

- A substance in the body that is normally strictly contained in a specific area (and thus is hidden from the immune system) is released into the general circulation. For example, the fluid in the eyeball is normally contained within the eyeball's chambers. If a blow to the eye releases this fluid into the bloodstream, the immune system may react against it.
- A normal body substance is altered. For example, viruses, drugs, sunlight, or radiation may change a protein's structure in a way that makes it seem foreign.
- The immune system responds to a foreign substance that is similar in appearance to a natural body substance and inadvertently targets the body substance as well as the foreign substance.
- Something malfunctions in the cells that control antibody production. For example, cancerous B lymphocytes may produce abnormal antibodies that attack red blood cells.

Is Endometriosis An Auto-Immune Disease?

*New research is showing that the health of our immune system can play
a major role in endometriosis. Some researchers are suggesting that
endometriosis may actually be an auto-immune disease.*

Is endometriosis a condition where the immune system is attacking the self? It seems true that an auto-immune reaction is taking place, when particles of the body are found in areas where they should not be i.e., the endometrium.

In the case of endometriosis, the immune system should be attacking those stray cells, but it is not clearing up the stray cells completely. It is left unchecked, which is why these stray cells go on to develop into endometriosis.

In women who do **not** have endometriosis, but who do have stray endometrial cells in the pelvic cavity, these stray cells are cleaned up by the immune system.

As mentioned earlier, a very high percentage of women do actually have retrograde menstruation which will contain endometrial cells, but because their immune system is functioning properly, then this debris is destroyed and not left in the pelvic cavity to go on and develop into endometriosis.

*No matter if endometriosis is an auto-immune disease, or
just the end result of a compromised immune system, it is
clear you need to support your immune system.*

Hippocratic Oath - Modern Version

If you have never read the Hippocratic Oath, I thought I would include it here for your reference – Point number two seems to be disregarded by many in medicine today. The insert in italics is from Wikipedia.

The Hippocratic Oath is an oath of ethics historically taken by physicians. It is one of the oldest and most widely known of Greek medical texts. In its original form, it requires a new physician to swear, by a number of healing gods, to uphold specific ethical standards. Different variations of the Hippocratic oath are taken by doctors around the world today.

I swear to fulfil, to the best of my ability and judgement, this covenant:

I will respect the hard-won scientific gains of those physicians in whose steps I walk, and gladly share such knowledge as is mine with those who are to follow.

I will apply, for the benefit of the sick, all measures which are required, avoiding those twin traps of over treatment and therapeutic nihilism.

(Therapeutic nihilism is a contention that it is impossible to cure people or societies of their ills through treatment. In medicine, it was connected to the idea that many "cures" do more harm than good, and that one should instead encourage the body to heal itself. Wikipedia)

I will remember that there is art to medicine as well as science, and that warmth, sympathy, and under-standing may outweigh the surgeon's knife or the chemist's drug.

I will not be ashamed to say "I know not," nor will I fail to call in my colleagues when the skills of another are needed for a patient's recovery.

I will respect the privacy of my patients, for their problems are not disclosed to me that the world may know. Most especially must I tread with care in matters of life and death. If it is given me to save a life, all thanks. But it may also be within my power to take a life; this awesome responsibility must be faced with great humbleness and awareness of my own frailty. Above all, I must not play at God.

I will remember that I do not treat a fever chart, a cancerous growth, but a sick human being, whose illness may affect the person's family and economic stability. My responsibility includes these related problems, if I am to care adequately for the sick.

I will prevent disease whenever I can, for prevention is preferable to cure.

I will remember that I remain a member of society, with special obligations to all my fellow human beings, those sound of mind and body as well as the infirm.

If I do not violate this oath, may I enjoy life and art, respected while I live and remembered with affection thereafter. May I always act so as to preserve the finest traditions of my calling and may I long experience the joy of healing those who seek my help.

Written in 1964 by Louis Lasagna, Academic Dean of the School of Medicine at Tufts University, and used in many medical schools today.

A FEW POINTS TO KEEP IN MIND ...

Many women have had success going the natural route

Your body is always striving to heal

There are many, many options you can try

Don't say 'I will get better' instead say '
I am getting better'

It's time to prioritize your health and needs

It's time to treat your whole body, not just your symptoms

This is a journey - not a race

Brief Outline To Your Healing Journey

Managing endometriosis naturally is about treating the whole body. It is about supporting your physical as well as emotional health. Getting results may mean trying different things because we are all different, our bodies are different, our immune systems are different and the length of time you have had this disease will also weigh in.

1. You need to stop putting bad stuff IN your body. You need to change to eating an anti-inflammatory diet and stop eating those foods with additives and zero nutrition. You also need to be eating nutrient dense foods that support your system and ensure a healthy gut microbiome.

2. Ideally you need to get rid of the bad stuff - change your toiletries, cosmetics and household cleaners for more natural options. These products contain many toxins and chemicals that can upset your natural hormones, making your endometriosis symptoms worse and can cause other health problems.

3. Aim to change your commercial period products for more natural options that do not contain chemicals. Most of these products contain a host of toxins and can really upset your hormones and your endocrine system. There are many natural period products available on the market you can use instead.

4. Try to get some gentle exercise. I know from personal experience this can be difficult but if you can manage a gentle walk or some simple yoga, this will help boost your endorphins (natural pain-killers) and will help to keep you more supple.

5. Do your best to get a good night's sleep. There are certain calming herbs you can use to help calm your system and help you sleep, as well as self-help calming measures you can use which we look at later in the book.

This is just the tip of the ice-berg of what we will be covering to support your health. We start by looking at different natural therapies that can help reduce your symptoms and support your body.

So let's begin ....

Natural

Treatments

for

Endometriosis

'Take care of your body.
It's the only place you have to live.'

Jim Rohn

Natural Treatments Introduction

Women with endometriosis are given few treatment options by their doctors. It usually includes painkillers, hormone therapy like birth control, surgeries, and a hysterectomy when all else fails. Surgery has been found to be a temporary fix at best which can then lead to even worse symptoms caused by more scar tissue. Drugs with their many side effects are also very damaging. Treating the body with kindness with natural therapies, diet, reducing toxins and supporting the immune system will reap better results for long term health.

Receiving treatment from any of the natural therapies available today can provide multiple benefits. You will have a targeted treatment plan specifically for you, and if you have additional health problems as well as endometriosis these can also be addressed. Additionally, you will often receive emotional support along with your treatment plan.

Natural treatments are defined more as a total holistic approach to healing rather than an isolated treatment. This method of treatment focuses on the person's whole being – physical, emotional, mental and spiritual. One of the primary benefits of natural therapies is they have few side effects, unlike modern drug treatments.

Surgical advances may be impressive but with endometriosis, all this does is remove the visible signs of the disease but does not treat the cause, and very often the disease can return after surgery. Whereas natural therapies aim to get to the root cause of disease and illness.

Getting support from a natural health therapist can be pivotal for many with endometriosis; to receive guidance and support as well as obtaining a specific treatment plan for their individual health needs. I feel my own healing would not have been as successful and total had I not had the support of my homeopath.

In hindsight it is difficult to ascertain whether I would have healed without this support, but I personally feel that having the ongoing support from someone who is working to fix your health, helps to feed into your confidence of being able to heal, and provides a safe place to have a sounding board through your healing journey. It was my own success with going the natural route for my endometriosis that prompted me to undertake my training in natural therapies, to help other women going through this ordeal.

It has been found that the very process of receiving care and being nurtured can be very instrumental in aiding the healing process. Just look how both people and animals respond to being in a supportive and caring environment. This is where problems can arise when those with endometriosis are living in a situation where they are not receiving the support they need from those around them.

Receiving treatment from any of the natural therapies provides a treatment plan that treats the whole body and aims to get to the route of the disease. Trying to do this on your own can be stressful especially when you do not know where to start, or worried if you are doing things right to support your health.

When choosing a natural therapy, you need to consider if the type of treatment is suitable for you. For example, are you happy taking herbal mixtures, or would you be OK with having needles stuck in you with acupuncture? Most importantly, you also need to feel comfortable and have confidence with the person you will be working with, as personalities can be just as important.

I am not saying it is imperative to see a natural therapist to obtain success, but I personally feel the added benefits of emotional support combined with safe natural treatments can aid in the whole healing package.

If you are unable to afford support from a natural therapist there is still so much you can do to heal your body, and one key support to healing is through gut health and nutrition combined with reducing toxins in your system. We go into these topics in some depth further on in the book.

Let's dive into the different natural therapies, which may help you choose which particular natural treatment you wish to use.

> 'By cleansing your body on a regular basis and eliminating as many toxins as possible from your environment, your body can begin to heal itself, prevent disease, and become stronger and more resilient than you ever dreamed possible.'

> - Dr. Edward Group

Acupuncture

Acupuncture is part of Traditional Chinese Medicine and has been practised in China for thousands of years, but became widely known in the West only in the 1970s, when its use as an anaesthetic received sensational press coverage.

Practitioners insert fine, sterile needles into specific points on the body as a treatment for disorders ranging from asthma to alcohol addictions, but most often in the West as a means of pain relief.

Acupuncture is an element within the Traditional Chinese Medicine health system, which includes herbs, acupressure, exercise, and diet. Fundamental to Traditional Chinese Medicine are the concepts of yin and yang, opposite but complementary forces whose perfect balance within the body is essential for well-being.

Yin and yang are components of qi (also known as chi), which is the invisible 'life energy' that flows through meridians (channels) around the body. There are 12 regular meridians running up and down the body in 6 pairs. They are mostly named after the main internal organs through which they pass.

Consulting an Acupuncturist

On your first visit, the practitioner will take notes on your lifestyle and medical history, and assess your condition using the 'Four Examinations' of Traditional Chinese Medicine - asking, observing, listening and touching, in which the most important test is taking the pulse.

This is a skilled method of checking the rhythm and strength of all 12 meridian pulses. To aid diagnosis, the practitioner may examine other parts of the body. They will then discuss treatment options, which as well as acupuncture, often include advice on diet and lifestyle, and may involve herbs.

The treatment involves lying on a treatment couch, after removing any clothing covering the needle sites. The site depends on the disorder and whether the flow of qi is to be 'warmed', reduced or increased.

Several acupoints may be used, those on the hands and feet are often treated, but sites on the back, abdomen, shoulders, and face are also widely used.

The practitioner inserts the needles to a depth of 1/8th - 1 inch depending on the position of the acupoint being treated. A treatment often involves a combination of acupoints; usually 6 - 12 needles are used, varying according to the type of acupuncture and condition being treated.

Acupuncture needles may be left in position for a few minutes, as little as a few seconds, or as long as an hour. At the end of the session, they are withdrawn swiftly and gently, usually painlessly, without bleeding, and leave no trace on the skin.

Treatment times vary greatly, from 30 to 90 minutes, depending on how long the needles are left in position. The initial consultation will probably be the longest. Most conditions require between 10 to 20 sessions, depending on the patients age and how long they have been suffering from the condition.

A growing number of doctors now practise 'medical acupuncture', usually for pain relief. For pain relief, acupuncture may release painkilling endorphins. It may also trigger nerve 'gate control', in which pressure messages reach the brain faster than the messages of pain, but more research is needed in this area. Generally speaking, there seems to be a lot of success with acupuncture to relieve pain.

This particular benefit will obviously be of special interest to those who suffer lots of pain with endometriosis. It would be advisable to seek out an acupuncturist to discuss treatment to help with your pain, and you will gain added benefits as acupuncture can also help to support the immune-system.

I personally know of one acupuncturist who has successfully treated women with endometriosis, and had great success not only in reducing the pain, but also eliminating the disease for a number of women.

This was seen as a long-term plan of treatment, and like all alternative treatments, involved raising the levels of 'life energy', and in turn supporting the immune system to fight the disease.

Success with Acupuncture

'After 7 1/2 years of trying with all fertility options including in-vitro I gave up and a friend recommended Acupuncture for my horrible symptoms. I went for acupuncture for 2 months three times a week and she changed my cycle to where I did NOT have any symptom i.e., heavy bleeding cramping etc. and told me to try and conceive. We got pregnant the first month. Just another option which worked great for me. '

Herbalism

Herbal medicine is the treatment of disease using medicinal plants, both internally and externally, to help restore health. It is a system of medicine that relies on the therapeutic qualities of plants to help by enhancing the body's own recuperative powers. It is a natural method of healing based on the traditional use of herbs coupled with modern scientific developments.

Though there are those in the orthodox medical world who ignore herbal medicine, even condemn it, the constituents of herbs have provided the blueprint for many of the most effective and widely known drugs used today. Modern medicine has its roots in herbal medicine.

Modern orthodox medicine is based on drugs isolated from plants, or more often manufactured in the laboratory. The herbalist advocates the use of the whole plant as a gentler and safer way to restoring a patient to health.

All medicinal plants contain a range of different therapeutic agents and therefore have a variety of different actions, related to the combined effects of these components.

- They relax tissues or organs which are over tense, predominantly muscles and the nervous system
- They stimulate 'atonic' tissues or organs (those lacking tone) such as sluggish bowel or liver
- They cause constriction of over relaxed tissues, such as muscles, blood vessels and mucous membranes producing excessive catarrhal secretions
- They promote elimination of wastes and poisons from the liver, bowel, kidneys and skin. This particular action is of real benefit for endometriosis sufferers, to help eliminate toxins and unwanted estrogens

- They help overcome infection by stimulating the body's defences and also have direct antiseptic, antibiotic and anti-fungal actions
- They enhance the circulation of blood and lymph
- They aid appetite and digestion and stimulate the absorption and assimilation of nutrients from our diet
- They soothe mucous membranes and thereby reduce irritation and inflammation - another good benefit for endometriosis
- They regulate the secretion and action of hormones and where necessary promote hormone production - this action will benefit endometriosis by balancing the hormone levels
- Herbal remedies are less harmful than chemical drugs. However, it is a mistake to suppose that natural means completely safe in any amount. There are some herbs which must be treated with great respect and care. Some of these herbs can be toxic if taken incorrectly.

Consulting a Practitioner

You need to find a qualified Medical Herbalist and ideally, they should have been trained in all the basic medical sciences - physiology, anatomy, pathology and different diagnosis techniques. They should also have passed a theoretic as well as clinical exam in physical examination techniques and diagnosis. They will also have studied plant pharmacology.

The first session will take about an hour and subsequent visits about 15 to 30 minutes. Details of any conventional medication you are taking will also be recorded to ensure compatibility with the herbal remedies prescribed.

The practitioner will carry out some simple tests or give you a physical examination. Based on the practitioner's conclusions, you will be prescribed one or more herbal remedies. Treatment may also include advice on diet and exercise and life-style changes.

The active properties within certain plants have been used for endometriosis to provide relief from symptoms, to help the body detox, and to counteract the synthetic estrogens taken up by the body from pollutants and house-hold chemicals.

Success with herbalism

'After 13 years of having to take anti-inflammatory medications for my menstrual cycle, I was not able to function without them. After a ruptured ovary, surgery and extreme endometriosis, my options for a "normal" life involved taking the pill along with an experimental drug that would tell the body it was in menopause or pregnancy, or I could have a hysterectomy.

I used a herbal formula from my herbalist regularly for six weeks. I was two weeks late with my menstrual cycle, so I figured that the formulas were not working. To my surprise, when I did have my period, I didn't have to use any anti-inflammatory medication.

I experienced only one day of cramps that were about 1/10th of the severity that they normally were. Furthermore, I didn't become as sick with nausea or diarrhoea as I usually do.

I have been suffering with this problem for many years while thinking that it was never going to go away unless I had a hysterectomy. Certainly, at only age 26, that procedure held its own complications and repercussions! I am very grateful for the opportunity to try an alternative approach that really works! Thank you for my life back!'

Kirsty USA

Another success using herbalism

'I am extremely happy that I am able to share my story with those who are looking into alternative treatment for endometriosis. For seven long years I went from specialist to specialist, treatment after treatment, only to be told there was no hope for me. I was diagnosed with Endometriosis. I did not know what to do.

My marriage was falling apart. Then one day my co-worker told me about a local herbalist who was treating with herbs. At first, I thought herbs and fertility, what do they have in common? I was desperate so I went to see the herbalist.

After having had consultations and being given the herbs that were prescribed to me, I went home not convinced that would happen, but I tried. I had the notion that only medical professionals can help such a problem. To my surprise three months after my visit, I was pregnant. My family life changed drastically. My husband and I are happy raising our little boy. My message to those suffering from endometriosis is to never give up hope.'

Margaret, Amsterdam, Holland

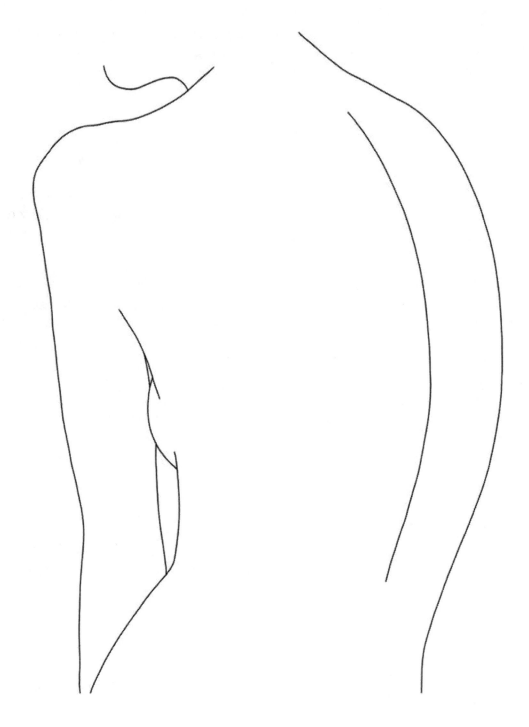

Naturopathy

Also known as 'Natural Medicine', naturopathy was developed in the late 19th century, founded on an ancient belief in the power of the body to heal itself. Naturopathy believes that the body's natural state is one of equilibrium, which can be disturbed by an unhealthy lifestyle. One of the key objectives of naturopathy is to get to the root cause of disease.

They look for underlying causes of a problem rather that treating symptoms alone, combining diet and non-invasive therapies where possible to stimulate the healing process. Naturopathy is practised throughout the Western world and some of its principles have been adopted by conventional medicine.

Modern naturopaths believe the body will always strive toward good health, or homeostasis, and that the body is its own best healer. They maintain that many factors, such as unhealthy diet, lack of sleep, exercise, or fresh air, any emotional or physical stress, pollution in the environment, even negative attitudes, allow waste products and toxins to build up in the body and upset self-regulation. This in turn can overload the immune system and weaken the vital force, the body's innate ability to maintain good health.

Naturopathic treatments are as non-invasive as possible. Some practitioners specialise in a particular approach, while others draw on a wide range of techniques. Some of the most commonly used treatments include nutrition and detoxing (diet is a very important part of naturopathic medicine).

Other treatments include physical therapies, including osteopathy, counselling and lifestyle modification. Additional treatments that may be offered include herbal medicine, homeopathy, Traditional Chinese Medicine, touch therapies including massage, acupressure, shiatsu, and yoga.

The training of the Naturopath will influence which treatments are offered. A naturopath will often work alongside other medical professionals you are currently working with to ensure a safe 'joined-up' treatment plan.

The whole approach with Naturopathy is totally holistic and covers many therapies and support techniques to aid good health and healing. Naturopaths use a variety of tests to assess the patients' health to build up a complete picture. This may include blood tests, testing for food sensitivities, salivary testing for hormones and testing for heavy metals and toxins.

Consulting a Practitioner

A naturopath works similarly to other therapists and will do a detailed questionnaire of your medical history and your lifestyle. The practitioner will then give you a routine medical examination, including tests on your blood pressure, lungs and heart, spinal joints and reflexes.

Treatment is aimed at building up a weakened constitution with nutritional supplements and changes to diet. The practitioner may give advice about breathing patterns, exercise and relaxation. Some naturopaths are also trained in counselling skills, and can assist in helping to manage the mental and emotional impact of illness.

Advice is tailored to individual needs, and willing participation in treatment and a positive mental attitude are crucial. Your health should improve steadily, possibly with temporary relapses known as the 'healing crisis' as detoxification takes effect. *We will be looking at the healing crisis further on.*

The Key Naturopathic Principles

- Work to restore and support the powerful healing ability of the body to prevent disease
- Identify the underlying cause, evaluating the root cause on all levels
- Seek to do no harm by employing safe, natural therapies
- Look at the whole health picture of the person and prepare a bespoke plan
- Educate and encourage the client to take responsibility for their own health
- Remove toxic substances and situations from a person's lifestyle to prevent and avoid further harm
- Establish and maintain optimal health by supporting the whole body to promote wellness
- Prevention is better than cure

Success with Naturopathy

'It is easy to feel a victim, not in the least because my GP couldn't really help me with my endometriosis. It was making my life hell and my husband was at his last tether. Undaunted and in the profound belief that all illnesses can be cured I sought Naturopathic help.

I was given a new dietary regimen of no dairy, meat, or eggs, and no white refined products such as pasta, white bread, and white rice. No ready-made meals. I had to learn how to cook properly. We eat plenty of fresh organic vegetables and whole grains foods now.

Yes my husband supported the diet change all the way. I was given herbs to cleanse and detox the body, particularly the liver, and to regulate my menstrual cycle. My Naturopath told me most gynaecological problems stem from liver imbalance.

My condition improved fabulously, which was very noticeable with each month. My overall health is now better than ever and completely clear of the former condition. I am so impressed I am taking up the study of Naturopathy to help others.'

Catherine

'With a few dietary and lifestyle changes, supplements, as well as herbal support, it can be managed very successfully. I myself have had endometriosis since I was 24. I had emergency surgery and hormone therapy, but later refused to have a hysterectomy! When I finally talked with Naturopathic doctors and Herbalists, I found out so much more about this condition, that none of the doctors I had seen were even aware of.

I adjusted my diet, took an herbal combination for several months, and went from to severe pain, to completely normal, pain-free cycles ever since! It has been over 8 years now, and I have had NO return of symptoms! My periods are great, I am happy and doing what I love!'

Cherie

'Apart from the pain, things went wrong when I was 20 - I bled for three months - non-stop. The doctor prescribed a high dosage contraceptive pill. The bleeding stopped but the pain continued. Eight years later Endo was diagnosed & Primulot prescribed. The pain went away (for a while) - that was wonderful.

My mood improved out of sight - terrific! I gained weight which I could not shift - that was not wonderful. The pain returned and the weight stubbornly remained. Twelve years on, I found a Naturopath and Herbalist who makes individual prescriptions; over a few months, the pain went away (that was wonderful) - and my energy improved (bonus!).'

Suzanne

Homeopathy

Homeopathy is a therapeutic method of medicine in which very dilute doses of natural substances (plant, animal, mineral) are administered to a patient to treat symptoms that would be induced in a healthy individual by ingestion of that same substance.

Homeopathy stimulates the body's own defences to correct illness and allow symptoms to dissipate. The minute doses of drug substances used in homeopathy do not cause any side effects. Homeopathy can be used for short term (acute) illnesses and long term (chronic) illnesses.

The healing method of homeopathy looks at each patient and develops a remedy or treatment plan strictly for him or her. It invokes the powers of healing inherent in individuals (our immune system) to develop a successful therapy. The more one knows about the patient, the symptoms, likes and dislikes, what makes them better or worse, the more it helps in developing a 'symptom picture' of the patient that can lead to a successful treatment.

Acute symptoms such as pain, heavy bleeding, mood swings, bloating, pre-menstrual symptoms and bowel upsets can be treated effectively with what is called an acute remedy. These can replace the need for painkillers, laxatives, sedatives and anti-depressants. Some examples of commonly used acute remedies are Magnesium Phosphate, Camomile, Helonias, Sepia and Cimicifuga.

There are over *400 different remedies for abdominal pain*, each one being quite specific to include: location of pain, length of pain, type of pain, time of day of worse pain, and so on. This is why it is not advisable to self-treat, and you need treatment from a qualified Homeopath for accurate remedies to be prescribed.

Consulting a Practitioner

Practitioners may be homeopaths who are not medically qualified or conventional doctors who practise homeopathy. The practitioner will ask you about your medical history, diet, lifestyle, moods, likes and dislikes, as well as the medical history of the problem you are seeking help for. A classical homeopath will also identify your 'constitutional type'.

The 'constitutional type' is identified through a person's individual physical, intellectual and emotional traits. This is done by asking many questions about your habits, fears, food preferences, personality attributes, the way different weather and seasons affect you. By doing this, homeopaths can prescribe remedies for the ailment and other remedies to support the person's constitutional type.

The practitioner will try to match your symptom picture with those catalogued in the homeopathic 'repertories', which include 2,000 to 3,000 remedies, often stored on a computer database. The skill lies in prescribing the remedy that fits your individual type and condition. Advice about diet and lifestyle may also be given.

You will be asked to report any reactions and changes in symptoms at your next visit, and your prescription may be altered or adjusted as necessary. With self-limiting conditions, practitioners say that improvement should occur after the first few doses of the correct remedy. Long-term conditions that have developed gradually require longer treatment, and can take many months. Once signs of improvement show, the remedy dose may be tapered off and eventually discontinued. A variety of remedies may be used in complex cases.

There are no side-effects with homeopathy, but symptoms may briefly worsen after treatment, which is something I suffered during my treatment for endometriosis. Homeopaths claim that since the body is healed from the inside out, deep-seated conditions may be temporarily replaced by more superficial ones. For example, as asthma improves, eczema may flare up in its place.

Success with Homeopathy

A success story from a surgical doctor who later trained to become a homeopath

Jane started her career in conventional medicine, managing one of the busiest hospital operating theatres in London. When she fell ill, conventional medicine failed her. In desperation she went to a homeopath, who cured her of her endometriosis. She was so impressed that she trained as a homeopath while she was still running the operating theatres of the hospital, eventually leaving to become a full-time practitioner herself.

'Homeopathy is a complementary medicine. It works on its own, and also with other medical treatments, be they conventional, or alternatives like Alexander therapy, reflexology or cranial osteopathy. I treat people holistically, encouraging them to appreciate the importance of tackling health with nutritional improvements as well as using homeopathy.

Increasingly I have to treat patients who come to me quite ill after extreme regimes of antibiotics or steroids or other toxic drugs. I believe that homeopathy is probably one of the most evolved and effective methods of healing, because it doesn't just treat, it cures. It is very understandable that its growing in popularity and successes are causing the pharmaceutical companies some concern.'

More success with homeopathy

'Mrs T. came with endometriosis and excruciating back, stomach and period pains, and was due to have a hysterectomy. The first treatment brought some relief from the pains, but she also experienced stomach bloating and carpal tunnel in her left wrist (she had had this ten years before - return of old symptoms).

Over the next 9 months there were many changes - the bloating and the pain disappeared, but headaches and depression returned. The headaches then disappeared, but she had terrible sciatica for a while. Then period pains stopped. One year later they returned with a vengeance, but after one treatment they disappeared and she was finally free from pain. One very exciting result - the consultant changed her mind about the hysterectomy - she said an operation was no longer necessary!'

13

Traditional Chinese Medicine

Traditional Chinese Medicine (TCM) views endometrial lesions as static blood – blood that is not flowing as it should, thus causing problems. TCM looks at the symptoms and signs that characterise an individual woman's disease, identifying patterns that give clues as to the underlying imbalance, or root cause, of the disease. A treatment plan is then tailored to the individual.

In Traditional Chinese Medicine diagnosis is made based on symptoms and categorized based on eight principles (yin and yang, empty and full, etc).

Two women, both experiencing endometriosis, may be diagnosed differently based on their symptoms – where and when pain occurs, colour and texture of menstrual blood, aggravating and relieving factors, and other signs. Naturopathic Doctors are often trained in TCM diagnosis and will individualize treatment plans for their patient based on their unique symptoms and experience of endometriosis.

When determining the pattern of disease, TCM takes into account the menstrual history, duration of the cycle, as well as pain, including the time that it occurs, the location, and the nature and severity.

In TCM theory, there are several disease-causing factors including blood stagnation, energy stagnation and deficiency, as well as cold and heat conditions that can lead to endometriosis. The origin of the pattern differs according to the individual.

Other factors that are taken into consideration when determining the pattern for disease include: emotional stress, anxiety, constitutional weakness, surgical history, exposure to cold temperatures especially during menstruation, diet, chronic illness or weakness, or a history of genital infections.

Treatments used with Traditional Chinese Medicine

Chinese Medicine uses a range of treatments such as Acupuncture, Cupping and Moxibustion along with herbal supplements and teas. The effect of these can be enhanced by lifestyle changes.

Nutritional Therapy is also important for those suffering with endometriosis. Chinese medicine encourages the body to produce natural anti-inflammatory compounds through proper nutrition. As the liver is responsible for detoxifying excess estrogen, foods that support the liver will be recommended, in order to naturally decrease estrogen levels.

As with other natural therapies, TCM provides alternative drug free treatment for those suffering with endometriosis, without side effects.

Success with Chinese Medicine and Acupuncture

In a letter to the Endometriosis Association, one patient wrote:

'Several years ago, I was fortunate enough to be pointed toward Edie Vickers, the acupuncturist associated with the Institute for Traditional Medicine in Portland, Oregon. At the time, I was adamant that under no circumstances would I subject myself to Danazol.

Through regular acupuncture and Chinese herbal treatments, I was able to delay my second endometriosis surgery for a year and a half, at which time the technology and knowledgeable and experienced doctor were available to take care of the majority of my problem via surgical technique.

At this time I was 37 years old...I am now 41 years old and consider myself lucky that I still have my uterus, have never taken Danazol or Lupron, and my pain is reduced to only needing ibuprofen - relieved cramps lasting no longer than 18 hours a month ... I think the herbs are greatly helpful and I always felt they were really working well. Chinese medicine takes patience, faith, and time, and sometimes lifestyle changes ... but, in the final analysis, it works.'

Nutritional Therapy

Nutritionists are trained in understanding the scientific base of nutrition and can provide insights into how the food we eat impacts on our health and well-being, based on science and facts. You will find there are different titles for nutritionists in addition to various levels of training and qualifications. As well as having relevant training, having experience can sometimes be more important, and having knowledge of a particular health problem can help the therapist have a deeper understand of the issues involved.

Working with a nutritionist can assist on many fronts regarding diet, gut health, checking for deficiencies as well as helping to monitor your progress. Essentially, a nutritionist knows how food affects our health on a deep level.

Using nutrition to help with endometriosis has gained a lot of credibility and there are now a number of nutritionists who specialise in providing advice for women with endometriosis, many of whom are dealing with the disease themselves. Having personally experienced the immense benefits of using nutrition to help with endometriosis, nutrition has been a corner-stone of my own training to help other women, along with training in natural therapies.

Seeing a Nutritionist

Before seeing a nutritionist, you will probably be asked to fill in a health questionnaire along with a detailed food diary for at least three days, but a seven-day food diary will provide a more detailed insight into your current eating habits.

The health questionnaire will probably cover:
- Details of reason for seeing the therapist/nutritionist
- Your current symptoms
- Medical history including surgeries
- Medications you are taking
- Supplements you are taking
- Digestion/bowel habits
- Your family history
- Energy levels
- Sleep habits
- Levels of exercise/ physical activity
- Lifestyle/ typical routine
- Toxin exposure

After returning your diet and health questionnaire you will then be able to make your initial appointment with the therapist.

You will then be guided on diet changes to make and possible tests that may be needed to assess any gut health problems like Leaky gut, SIBO, histamine intolerances etc. If you have any particular gut health problems then a specific treatment regime will be compiled. Advice about the addition of any supplements will also be provided often based on the outcome of testing. Your treatment regime will continue which will be tailor made for you, and will include ongoing assessments to check for the need of any changes that need to be made.

Depending how serious the level of disease will often determine how long you need to see a nutritionist, but very often women start to see improvements within the first few months. Once improvements start to be noticeable you will be able to lengthen the time between appointments.

Pelvic Floor Physical Therapy

Pelvic Floor Therapy involves exercises and stretches that help to strengthen and relax the pelvic floor. Pelvic Therapy can help to manage the symptoms of endometriosis such as painful menstrual cramping, abdominal discomfort, pelvic floor pain, and painful intercourse.

This is achieved by:
- treating connective tissue dysfunction
- treating myofascial trigger points
- gentle manual therapy techniques aimed at releasing adhesions and restoring the proper mobility of the internal organs, such as the uterus, bladder, colon and small intestine
- correcting postural and movement dysfunction

You need to be aware that having Pelvic Floor Physical Therapy involves internal examination, which some may find emotionally uncomfortable. During the internal exam, your physical therapist will place a gloved finger into your vagina or rectum to assess the tone and strength of your pelvic floor muscles and tissues.

These internal exams can tell if there are trigger points (painful spots), muscle/tissue shortening, or nerve irritation and/or bony malalignment that could be causing pain directly or inhibiting the full function of your pelvic floor muscles.

Exercises and massage are used to release trigger points and muscles are aligned, and you may be given exercise to perform at home. A therapist may teach you exercises of how to contract and relax pelvic floor muscles in relation to other muscles. You may also be taught breathing and timing techniques to make the exercises more effective. Such exercises can stretch tight muscles, strengthen weak ones, and improve flexibility.

Many are having success using this particular therapy to help reduce their symptoms, but like I said, it depends how you feel about having internal manipulation and treatment.

Natural Therapies Summary

As you can see there are various natural and alternative therapies available, all of which will provide a treatment plan specific to you. There are many other therapies not covered here, each having very specific means of treatment and diagnosis.

The instincts you have about a therapy or a practitioner are important, as belief and trust play a significant role in healing. Make sure that your practitioner is reputable and suitably trained.

You are likely to respond better to a therapy if its principles fit with your ideas on well-being and if you feel comfortable with its approach. This was how I arrived at my own choice of which natural therapy to use.

Issues to consider about the type of therapy to use include:

- are you happy about being touched or having a massage?
- are you OK about swallowing pills and can usually remember to take them regularly?
- are you comfortable exploring your feelings with another person?
- would you be prepared to change your diet radically?
- can you tolerate the idea of having needles stuck in you?
- are you comfortable about the practitioner manipulating your body?

Before embarking on any course of therapy you should ask your practitioner these questions:

- What are the practitioners' qualifications? What sort of training was undertaken, and for how long?
- How many years has the practitioner been in practise?
- Is treatment available on referral by your doctor? Some therapies, such as chiropractic, osteopathy and acupuncture, are becoming accepted into mainstream medicine.
- Can you claim for the treatment through your health insurance?
- What is the cost of treatment?
- How many treatments might you expect to require?
- Can treatment be done by Zoom and various remote methods?

I will repeat, trust and empathy with your practitioner are important, and treatment success may be reduced without it. Treatment is conducted on a one-to-one basis, so you need to feel comfortable with the person you work with.

Healing and managing endometriosis naturally is about being comfortable with the treatment plan you are undertaking. You have a number of options available and there is no need to rush before deciding which treatment to use.

As with any treatment plan and lifestyle changes, it can take at least 6-12 months of being consistent to bring about real change in the body when living with endometriosis. So don't give up when things get tough, I promise that these changes will be worth it in the long run!

A great story which emphasis the benefit of a multi-discipline approach

'Within the last year I finally figured out that what I've been experiencing all my life was endo. I'm 37. My mom had it so bad that she had a total hysterectomy in her 20's. I think one of the reasons I didn't suspect endo was that my mom was so used to bad periods that she told me mine were normal.

Anyway, things were getting so bad that I was having to take like 3 days off of work each period and almost passing out on my worst day. Then once my period is over, I experience this pain that I can only describe as if my uterus was coming detached.

Things I've tried...

Went from tampons to reusable pads. - This helped decrease the intensity of my cramps. I recently had to use tampons while swimming and the difference was really noticeable in my cramp pains.

Made sure I was getting enough omega-3 fatty acids. Started taking fish oil then just tried to make diet changes that included them. This has been the biggest change so far. I went from overdosing on ibuprofen every period to taking no ibuprofen.

Started eating paleo-diet (I'm not super strict because I love real yogurt and certain cheeses). That took my period down to 2 days of blood and light cramps. I still get 5 days of spotting beforehand but if there is no pain, I don't care.

Next, I went to a naturopath because I am still experiencing the weird post period pain. He has me on Maca root and suggested some other herbs. He also had me go off of coffee and alcohol for a while. He said endo is an estrogen dominance problem and both of those substances are estrogenic.

I'm just now going to natural deodorants and body products and am seriously considering banning plastics and chemicals from our house to see if that has an effect. My understanding is that all these unnatural substances are estrogenic.

Making these changes has really helped my symptoms and I am glad that things are now improving. I am glad I found the website at endo-resolved which is where I found the advice about the things that can make endometriosis worse. Making the few diet changes has made a big difference and I may try to make a few more changes in my diet.' - Jessica, UK

Aromatherapy Benefits

Essential oils can help with physical as well as mental health problems and can also be used in natural beauty treatments, which makes them valuable to have in your health tool-kit.

Essential oils need to be used with the same respect as prescription medication. Using the wrong oils for the wrong person can cause a negative reaction.

In an aromatherapy treatment, essential oils interact with the body in a variety of ways. When massage oil is prepared with essential oils and rubbed on the skin, the essential oils are quickly absorbed through the cell tissue and into the bloodstream to be transported throughout the body. They can then interact with the organs and systems of the body directly.

Scientists working in a number of different fields around the world have carried out laboratory tests which prove that essential oils have the ability to prevent the spread of harmful bacteria. Most essential oils have antibiotic, antiseptic, anti-viral and anti-inflammatory properties to a greater or lesser extent.

Properties of different oils

Stimulating oils

(for low blood pressure and lack of energy)

Basil, black pepper, cardamom, ginger, peppermint, pine needle, rosemary, thyme

Relaxing oils

(for emotional or physical tension)

Cedarwood, bergamot, camomile, clary-sage, cypress, frankincense, jasmine, lavender, neroli, rose, sandalwood, ylang ylang

Anti-inflammatory/Healing oils

(especially beneficial for endometriosis sufferers)

Benzoin, bergamot, camomile, frankincense, geranium, lavender, myrrh, patchouli, rose

Anti-spasmodic oils

(for period pains, muscle cramps)

Black pepper, cardamom, camomile, clary sage, fennel, ginger, jasmine, lavender, marjoram, nutmeg, orange, rosemary

Anti-depressant oils

Basil, benzoin, bergamot, geranium, jasmine, lavender, neroli, petitgrain, rose, ylang ylang

You will note that many oils have more than one benefit

Some of the best essential oils for endometriosis are the ones that have anti-inflammatory and anti-spasmodic properties. There are other benefits to using essential oils for endometriosis including:

- help with insomnia and aid sleep
- relaxing oils to help with stress
- using anti-depressant oils
- detoxifying - to assist the release of toxins from the system
- relieve pre-menstrual tension

Aromatherapy can help ease the symptoms of endometriosis in a variety of ways. A really beneficial way is to use oils in bath water, having a soak last thing at night, adding oils that aid with sleep and relaxation.

When buying essential oils, always purchase high quality oils, and aim to purchase oils that are organic and keep them stored in a cool, dark place.

Over the years I have found aromatherapy to be very beneficial for both health and beauty purposes. For those women who want to stop using commercially produced body and face creams and reduce their use of chemicals, you can easily make your own preparations using essential oils. I personally use Almond oil as a base oil, then add whatever essential oils I wish to use at the time to make up an essential oil blend.

Essential oils can be used in the following ways:

- mixed with a carrier oil for massage and pain relief
- added to bath water for relaxation
- added to a carrier oil for a therapeutic body and face oil
- burned in a vaporiser so that the essential oils are vaporised in the atmosphere - good for colds and flu

Essential Oils For Endometriosis

Here are some of the best oils to help with endometriosis symptoms

Clary Sage - This heady and calming oil has many benefits for endometriosis.

Nervous system - this essential oil works by reducing tension, depression, stress and is really good for insomnia. Balance hormones - clary sage essential oil helps balance hormones and has been found to reduce the symptoms of endometriosis. Add 3 to 4 drops to some carrier oil and apply to your abdomen.

Note - Clary sage is often suggested to help with menstrual pain, but this oil can cause problems for some as it affects muscle contractions and can make period pain worse which is an issue for those with endometriosis. So, avoid using during your period to be safe.

Frankincense and Myrrh - When used in combination, these two essential oils work in synergy to help ease reproductive issues including endometriosis. The boswellic acid in frankincense oil has a similar action to NSAIDS (Nonsteroidal Anti-Inflammatory Drugs), but without the unwanted side effects!

Peppermint - Peppermint is a fresh smelling essential oil that contains menthol – a powerful compound that helps numb pain. Peppermint essential oil is a natural remedy for relieving menstrual cramps and can also support the liver by rubbing a few drops over the liver area.

Rosemary - This oil is good for promoting proper blood circulation and is often used in shampoos to promote blood circulation to the hair roots. Rosemary also has estrogen-balancing activity which helps balance your hormones.

For sore muscles bath blend: Combine: 1 drop of Copaiba, 1 drop of Peppermint and 3 drops of Frankincense with 1 tablespoon of Jojoba oil and 1/2 cup of Epsom salts. Stir together and add to running bath water for a relaxing soak.

Copaiba oil

This particular oil requires a special mention and many with endometriosis find this oil very helpful for pain and inflammation

Copaiba is considered to be one of the strongest anti-inflammatory substances available, and applied to the abdomen can provide much needed relief with inflammation and bloating with endometriosis.

Interestingly, not only does copaiba act as a pain killer, but it can also help reduce liver tissue damage caused by drugs like Tylenol. One study measured the effect of copaiba oil in liver damage that was induced by pain-killers in rats, and after 7 days it was found that the damage had been noticeably reduced. Copaiba can also help reduce scar tissue, and used with a carrier oil and rubbed over your abdomen, it will help to speed healing after surgery.

Benefits of Copaiba oil include:

- Eases pain
- Reduces inflammation
- Helps reduce scar tissue
- Speed wound healing
- Fights germs and infection
- Helps boost immunity
- Supports the nervous system
- Antibacterial
- Analgesic
- Antifungal
- Expectorant
- Anti-depressant properties

This oil blends really well with frankincense for pain relief, and needs to be diluted with a carrier oil – mix 5 drops with 10ml of carrier oil. You can also add a few drops to your bath water, and used in the evening will help relax you for a good night's rest.

Gut Health

&

Liver Detox

> *'When diet is wrong medicine is of no use,*
> *when diet is correct medicine is of no need'*
>
> *Ancient Ayurvedic Proverb*

What Can Go Wrong With The Gut?

Before going into details about diet and nutrition we first look at some possible gut health concerns that may be causing you problems.

Many with endometriosis appear to suffer a variety of gut health problems. Some of these issues are caused by the disease especially when it infiltrates the digestive system, while other problems can be side-effects of drugs, gut imbalances or food intolerances. You need to get on top of these gut problems otherwise any chance of recovering your health will be undermined.

Gluten/wheat intolerance or allergy - gluten intolerance is divided into three distinct categories: Celiac Disease, Non-Celiac Gluten Sensitivity and Wheat Allergy. Many women with endometriosis become very sensitive to gluten which can exacerbate their symptoms.

Leaky Gut - Leaky gut is just what it sounds like and the lining of your gut has become compromised and damaged which leads to your gut becoming permeable – in a word your gut is leaky. This means particles of food can pass through your gut wall and into your blood stream causing many nasty symptoms.

Small Intestinal Bacterial Overgrowth - this is where the balance of the gut becomes out of whack and you have too many bacteria in your small intestines. The symptoms can sometimes be confused with endometriosis and if left unchecked can lead to serious nutritional deficiencies.

Irritable Bowel (IBS) - the medical profession does not actually know what causes Irritable Bowel, but stress has been highlighted as the main trigger and many with endometriosis suffer IBS.

Candida - candida is a yeast overgrowth of the intestines but many doctors do not understand what causes this overgrowth, but stress and a compromised immune-system have been noted to be possible causes.

Possible Reasons For A Damaged Gut!

There are many reasons why you may have a damaged gut, and you may need to work on healing your digestive system

Bowel prep – usually taken before surgery for laparoscopy and colonoscopy. The powder that is prescribed gives the entire gut a thorough clean out – but it is so harsh it is like 'paint-stripper' for the gut. This will kill all the good bacteria in your gut and probably cause additional gut damage.

Drugs – on-gong long term use of painkillers can damage the gut. Narcotic pain relievers reduce the motility of stomach contents through the digestive tract. As foods move slower through the digestive tract, excess water is removed from the contents of the colon, which makes stools dryer, sometimes resulting in constipation.

Laxatives – trying to combat constipation with laxatives can damage your intestinal flora and cause damage to the lining of your intestines. They can also make the matter worse when laxative dependency develops.

Hormone drugs – can cause many side effects relating to gut health - abdominal swelling, nausea, gastro-intestinal upsets, and liver malfunction.

Stress – this is one key issue that can really upset the natural balance of digestive enzymes, it can suppress the digestive processes, can cause inflammation, decreases natural digestive secretions, and affects contractions of your digestive muscles.

You can see by the list above that you need to try and address these issues. The use of drugs can damage the gut possibly causing Leaky Gut, SIBO and additional gut problems. By reducing your use and dependency on painkillers, laxatives, and hormone drugs you will put less stress on your gut as well as your liver.

Leaky Gut And Endometriosis

Leaky Gut can cause symptoms that may be confused as symptoms of endometriosis and many with endometriosis seem to suffer from leaky gut.

Dr. Shanti Mohling who is a gynaecological surgeon and researcher at the University of Tennessee, whose research is funded by the Endometriosis Foundation, has noticed a correlation between intestinal permeability, commonly known as leaky gut and the presence of endometriosis.

Leaky gut, or "intestinal permeability," is a condition in which the lining of the small intestine becomes damaged, causing undigested food particles, toxic waste products and bacteria to "leak" through the intestines and flood the blood stream.

The lining of your intestines is only one cell thick and these intestinal cells form the barrier, known as the gut barrier that separates the gut from the rest of the body. This gut barrier contains 'gates' that open and close to let nutrients get through. These 'gates' are actually tight junctions between each of the cells of your gut lining.

Certain foods can trigger leaky gut, especially gluten, dairy and soy as they can be seen as foreign invaders by the body. Leaky gut can also be caused by certain medication including anti-biotics, steroids and OTC pain medications like aspirin which can irritate the gut lining.

Leaky gut can lead to leaky brain

I am not trying to be alarmist here, but simply want to make you aware of the diverse possible symptoms related to having a leaky gut. The gut and the brain, as we are learning, are closely connected, and poor gut health can lead to poor brain health and related symptoms. This is called the brain-gut axis.

Leaky gut is related to 'leaky brain,' in which the blood-brain-barrier, a protective membrane around the brain, becomes compromised. This allows pathogens to enter the brain, leading to inflammation of the brain and symptoms of brain fog, which is commonly reported by women with endometriosis. Other symptoms can include fatigue, anxiety and poor memory.

Leaky gut has also been shown to play a role in depression by allowing harmful bacteria into the bloodstream. These bacteria carry large molecules that trigger inflammatory cytokines. Once in the bloodstream these bacteria cause inflammation throughout the body. These inflammatory cytokines also activate the brain's immune system, creating brain inflammation and degeneration, altering how well neurons function and communicate. This can ultimately change brain function and cause severe depression.

Symptoms of Leaky Gut

Some of the signs of leaky gut include having digestive issues of gas, diarrhoea, bloating and digestive upset. Suffering severe fatigue or muscle pain can also be additional clues. You may also suffer from food allergies which can trigger a worsening of symptoms.

Other symptoms can include headaches, joint pain, bowel issues, anxiety, sugar and carb cravings, nutrient deficiencies and hormone imbalances.

If you are looking to get tested for Leaky Gut, ask your practitioner for an intestinal permeability test, also known as the lactulose–mannitol challenge. This test measures how quickly the sugars lactulose and mannitol cross the lining of the gut.

It may not be necessary to do testing and you can take control of Leaky Gut through diet changes and healing your gut with supplements which we cover next. But this is something you should decide for yourself with medical guidance. Additionally, if your doctor is unwilling to do testing and you are looking to get private tests, these can be very expensive.

Treating Leaky Gut

The key to healing leaky gut is to change your diet and eliminate foods that the body may treat as toxic. Ensure you do not eat any gluten as this can aggravate the problem and can damage the gut lining. Also cut right back on sugar, which you should be doing anyway.

The main foods advised to omit for leaky gut include:

- Wheat
- Gluten
- Junk foods
- Dairy products
- Refined oils
- Baked items like cakes, cookie and pastries
- Soy, dressings and sauces

Adding healthy fats can help to heal a leaky gut such as oily fish, coconut oil and olive oil. Certain supplements that are helpful include collagen, N-acetyl Glucosamine as well as taking probiotics to restore healthy gut bacteria. There is a detailed list of gut healing supplements further on.

Collagen to heal a Leaky gut

Supplementing with collagen can really help leaky gut as it repairs the gut lining. You can supplement using collagen powder, and there are various products available on the market, but ensure you buy a reputable product.

The best type of collagen for gut health is a multi-blend containing collagen types 1, 2 and 3 to obtain the best benefits. The most common type of collagen is type 1 which helps hair, skin nails and bone health. Type 2 helps build cartilage, support gut lining health and aids immune function. Type 3 supports skin and bone health as well as supporting cardiovascular health.

Collagen is sourced from beef and chicken as well as fish and is available in powder form and capsules but the best type for maximum absorption is liquid collagen. Ensure the product you purchase is natural and free of pesticides, hormones and chemicals.

You can also obtain collagen from bone broth; however, it can prove too much trouble to be making up bone broth soup on a regular basis, and using a collagen supplement is an easier option.

Possible Histamine Reaction

For women with histamine sensitivity, taking collagen is usually not recommended as it can trigger a host of histamine intolerance symptoms. To be able to obtain the benefits of collagen to heal your gut without triggering a histamine reaction, taking histamine calming supplements at the same time will help to alleviate this reaction. These supplements include quercetin, bromelain and DOA (Diamine oxidase). Certain DOA supplements also contain vitamin C and quercetin to increase effectiveness – *we cover more on the topic of histamines further on.*

Colostrum for Leaky Gut

The supplement of colostrum is another really good option to help heal the gut. The growth factors in colostrum play a key role in correcting intestinal permeability. By stimulating cell growth, they strengthen the lining and improve the integrity of the gut.

Colostrum is extremely rich in antibodies that offer protection against disease-causing micro-organisms, including those in the gut. Colostrum also contains peptides that can regulate the immune-system. This is an important part of correcting leaky gut. When the immune system is working properly then inflammation can be controlled and the gut lining can heal.

Colostrum is found as a powder supplement as well as capsules and is readily available. However, if you are lactose intolerant then you need to avoid most colostrum products as it is obviously sourced from bovine milk. Fortunately, there is a specific colostrum formula, Colostrum-LD which is a lactose-reduced formula; lactase enzyme is added during processing to breakdown lactose making Colostrum-LD suitable for lactose-sensitive diets.

Small Intestinal Bacterial Overgrowth

As well as the possibility of having leaky gut, endometriosis sufferers can find themselves dealing with Small Intestine Bacterial Overgrowth.

- 84% of IBS cases are actually SIBO
- 50% of people with SIBO also have leaky gut

Small intestinal bacterial overgrowth (SIBO) is a serious condition affecting the small intestine. It occurs when bacteria that normally grow in other parts of the gut start growing in the small intestine. While bacteria naturally occur throughout the digestive tract, in a healthy system, the small intestine has relatively low levels of bacteria.

If left untreated it can lead to problems of malabsorption of nutrients, especially fat-soluble vitamins like vitamin A and D as well as iron. As women with endometriosis can easily become low in iron due to heavy periods, having depleted iron levels can make you feel very weak and fatigued.

Having a weakened immune system and abdominal surgery can be underlying causes of developing SIBO, as well as damage to the nerves and muscles of the gut can also increase your risk. Low stomach acid can be another risk factor along with a diet high in sugar and processed carbs.

SIBO symptoms mainly affect the gut

One of the notable symptoms is a bloated and distended stomach which may be mistaken as endo-belly, which in itself is very common. The bloating of SIBO is caused by gas produced from fermentation in the small intestine, triggered by the bacteria as it feasts on food in the gut. This process can build up as the day goes on and by the end of the day your belly can be very distended and painful accompanied by gas.

Other symptoms of SIBO include:
- Diarrhoea – usually associated with hydrogen dominant SIBO
- Constipation – usually associated with methane dominant SIBO
- Alternating constipation and diarrhoea
- Gas, flatulence, belching, severe bloating
- Abdominal pain and cramps
- Leaky gut – Intestinal permeability
- Weight loss or gain
- Food sensitivities
- Headache

- Chronic Fatigue Syndrome
- Fibromyalgia
- Lactose intolerance, Fructose intolerance, Sucrose intolerance
- Iron and B12 deficiency
- Fatigue
- Nausea

Getting tested

A breath test is one common test for diagnosing SIBO. Excess bacteria in the small intestine can lead to the release of the gases hydrogen and methane, which can be identified through a breath test. The test can be performed at home or at your doctor's office, which is done by drinking a special sugar solution.

The presence of hydrogen in the breath indicates bacteria are present in the small intestine as they interact with the sugar solution and releasing hydrogen or methane, which is then excreted through the breath. However, there is concern that these tests can return false-positive as well as false-negative results due to either fast or slow gut transit time.

You'll need to fast overnight before having a breath test. During the test, you'll breathe into a tube. You will then drink a special sweet drink provided by your doctor. You will breathe into a series of additional tubes at regular intervals for 2 to 3 hours after consuming the drink.

Other tests include a stool test and your doctor may request a blood test to check for nutrient deficiencies.

Treatment of SIBO

Antibiotics

The antibiotic Rifaxamin is considered the best antibiotic for hydrogen or Methane dominant SIBO and is often combined with neomycin which is an antibiotic that fights bacteria in the body.

Antimicrobials

A range of different natural plant-based antimicrobials have been found to be as effective against SIBO as the antibiotics and these can also impact on SIFO (small intestine fungal overgrowth).

Elemental Diet

The elemental diet involves consuming a drink that provides all of your daily nutrient needs but doesn't feed the bacteria. Studies show the elemental diet helps to eradicate SIBO in 85% of people.

By eliminating the need for the digestive system to perform normal digestive functions, as well as limiting the fuel source for bacteria, the elemental diet acts as a protective way to ensure that you still consume all the necessary nutrients. Also, during the treatment period it allows the bowels time to rest and decrease bacterial overgrowth.

You can find more details about the elemental diet here:

https://www.siboinfo.com/elemental-formula.html

Managing SIBO with herbal antimicrobials

As a nutritionist I recommend using herbs for SIBO and the use of antimicrobial herbs have been used very successfully. Some common herbs used in SIBO treatment include oil of oregano, allicin, berberine herbs, and neem. The treatment duration with herbal antimicrobials is typically longer than with antibiotics.

Berberine - consists of a compound found in Oregon grape, barberry, goldenseal, and other herbs.

Oregano - Oil of Oregano is a natural, powerful antibiotic, which is why it is often used to treat SIBO. Oregano oil is also use to treat candida.

Wormwood - Wormwood possesses several medicinal compounds which include anti-inflammatory, antimicrobial, and antioxidant properties. Wormwood can help in the treatment protocol for SIBO.

Indian Barberry Root - The bark of the trunk and root is known for its medicinal uses as it contains alkaloids that assist in a number of bodily functions, especially of the digestive track.

You need to work with a natural therapist for guidance to treating SIBO using herbal remedies, especially as SIBO can be difficult to treat.

To sum up

You need to be consistent with your treatment plan and then retest again. Sometimes it can take up to 3 to 4 rounds of treatment to get on top of SIBO as it can be a tough cookie to deal with. Untreated, SIBO can lead to chronic inflammation, gut issues, and the development of auto-immune conditions.

If you have been tested for SIBO and start treatment you may feel a bit rough with 'die-off' symptoms, but this usually only occurs if you are undergoing drastic treatment like taking potent anti-microbials or making big diet changes.

Symptoms will typically include flu-like symptoms, headache, brain-fog, constipation and digestive upset. This will pass as the treatment progresses and symptoms will gradually improve. Although these symptoms are not ideal, it is actually an indication that the treatment is working.

Just a couple of other points about managing SIBO is that prebiotics and probiotics may make SIBO worse. Additionally, consuming too much fibre can also cause problems as high fibre promotes more bacterial growth. This is because a high fibre diet can upset the balance in the gut causing excess fermentation in the large intestines, which can then spill over into the small intestines where all the trouble in your gut is taking place.

IBS & Endometriosis

Irritable Bowel Syndrome is another gut issue that can often occur with endometriosis. Research has found IBS is five times higher in women with endometriosis compared to women without the disease. However, it isn't fully understood why IBS is so common with this disease.

There seem to be certain contributing factors:

- The adhesions that occur with endometriosis (and surgery) can alter the structure of the digestive organs and can cause many of the symptoms associated with endometriosis and IBS.
- Both endometriosis and IBS are a chronic state of low-grade inflammation, which involves dysbiosis (an imbalanced microbiome) and increased intestinal permeability, otherwise known as Leaky Gut
- Stress is a major factor to consider in both conditions. Stress can affect gut motility, suppress the immune-system and increase gut inflammation.
- Low stomach acid is linked to SIBO and can interfere with the absorption of food.

How to manage IBS

It helps to work out your trigger foods that can set off an attack of IBS. If you are keeping a diary to monitor your symptoms then you should find it easier to find your triggers. Also, try to reduce your stress levels, as stress can really have a negative effect on the gut.

Unfortunately, it appears to be common to have both Small Intestinal Overgrowth (SIBO) along with IBS, and the estimate is two-thirds of those who test can have both of these digestive issues together.

IBS can be helped with supplements such as slippery elm and I am a great fan of aloe vera juice which is very healing for the gut. Probiotics such as lactobacillus plantarum and lactobacillus rhamnosus can also help. Lactobacillus rhamnosus is also thought to help with anxiety and depression as it supports GABA production (your calming neurotransmitter) in the brain.

Candida Albicans

This is yet another problem that can occur with endometriosis, and there is much speculation of there being a common link between Candida and endometriosis.

When immunity and resistance are low, the body loses its intestinal balance and Candida yeasts multiply too rapidly, feeding on sugars and carbohydrates in the digestive tract. Candida is often caused by a compromised immune system. Unless the body's weakened defences are given assistance, Candida colonies will flourish throughout the body and keep releasing toxins into the bloodstream.

Diet changes are a corner-stone to start managing Candida. The foods that should be eliminated with a diet for Candida are very similar to the foods that should be eliminated to deal with endometriosis. There are a few variations but the basics are the same.

For Candida, avoiding all forms of yeast forming foods, fermented foods, and mould foods is essential, as these will all help to feed the Candida yeast over-population. Candida albicans yeast normally lives harmlessly in the gastrointestinal tract and genito-urinary areas of the body. But Candida may infect virtually any part of the body.

If left unchecked Candida can infect deep internal organs, which can result in serious disease.

Lifestyle factors that promote Candida infection:

- Poor diet - especially excessive intake of sugar, starchy foods, yeasted breads and foods full of chemicals.
- Repeated use of antibiotics - long term use of antibiotics kill protective bacteria (which normally keep Candida under control).
- Hormone medications like corticosteroid drugs and birth control pills.
- High stress levels

Symptoms of Candida include:

- recurrent digestive problems, gas, bloating or flatulence
- rectal itching, or chronic constipation alternating to diarrhoea
- a white coating on your tongue (thrush)
- unusually irritable or depressed, unexplained frequent headaches, muscle aches and joint pain
- feel sick all over, yet the cause cannot be found.
- chronic vaginal yeast infections or frequent bladder infections
- psoriasis, eczema or chronic dermatitis
- catch frequent colds that take many weeks to go away

- oversensitive to chemicals, tobacco, perfume or insecticides.
- Crave sugar, bread or alcoholic beverages

Testing for Candida

It can prove challenging to obtain accurate tests for Candida. One of the reasons for this is that it is normal to find candida in the body. For this reason, it is common practise to look at multiple factors to test for candida overgrowth and yeast infection issues.

Tests for Candida may include:

Laboratory tests such as candida stool test, saliva test, blood test, urine test, candida antibodies test, vaginal discharge test.

Treating Candida

You need to stop eating foods that feed Candida and this includes all fermented foods, yeast foods, high sugar fruits, sugar including honey and molasses, processed and refined foods, soy, vinegars and condiments, pickled foods, gluten, processed meats, cheese and milk, refined oils, alcohol.

Natural remedies to treat Candida include:

- Probiotics especially Lactobacillus acidophilus
- Enteric coated capsules of Oregano oil or Peppermint oil
- Garlic – which can be taken as capsules

Making diet changes as suggested and adding supportive natural remedies as above will help to manage Candida overgrowth.

To Sum Up Gut Health Issues

IBS and SIBO are often the most common gut issues suffered by those with endometriosis, but don't assume you have any of these gut health problems just because you have endometriosis. Getting medical guidance and working with a specialist in gut health, or your doctor will help you get a correct diagnosis. This will then be supported by an appropriate treatment plan.

If you wish to take a natural route, these are the self-help measures you can take to heal your gut:

- Leaky gut can be managed with diet changes and using specific nutrients to heal the gut
- If you want to go the natural route, SIBO can be managed with natural antimicrobials and diet as we have covered
- For IBS it will help to find your trigger foods and an elimination diet will uncover your particular food triggers
- Candida can be managed by removing specific foods from you diet and supported with natural remedies

There are details of the Elimination diet further on, as well as a comprehensive list of supplements that can help heal the gut. Including digestive enzymes in your treatment regime will also support your digestive system and help you absorb vital nutrients, which is another topic we cover further on.

A short message of motivation ...

Focus on one thing at a time rather than trying to fix everything all at once.
Changing your lifestyle is a marathon, not a sprint.
You will have slip ups and that's okay.
Small steps lead to the bigger picture of the goal you want to achieve.

The Importance Of Your Gut Microbiome

There is a strong correlation between gut health and overall health as we are learning – this includes physical, mental as well as emotional health. A well-known naturopathic saying for good health is, 'First, heal the gut'. Your gut is the corner-stone of your health and well-being.

Reasons for needing a healthy gut:

1 The gut is home to the largest population of microbes living in our body and we suspect that these microbes drive our health in more ways than we currently understand. Science is just starting to understand the importance of the 'microbiome'. We depend on a vast army of microbes to stay alive: a microbiome protects us against germs, breaks down food to release energy, and helps produce vitamins and nutrients.

2 The gut is the foundation of our immune system, with approximately 80% of our immune tissue located in the digestive tract. Compromised gut health will mean our immunity deteriorates. You need a vibrant immune-system to help manage endometriosis and supporting the health of your gut will help to get to the route-cause of many gut-health problems we have just covered. If left unchecked these digestive imbalances can cause long-term distressing symptoms.

3 Gut health directly affects our hormone balance by affecting how certain hormones are metabolized and eliminated - and in some cases, influencing how hormones are produced. In women, we have something called the 'estrobolome' which impacts how estrogen is metabolized in the body which is a crucial factor in endometriosis.

4 Gut health not only affects how hormones are produced, but also has an effect on neurotransmitter production including serotonin and dopamine which are our feel-good chemicals – we will cover more on this later.

'If you have survived this far, well done! We are almost done dealing with gut health problems.'

Gut Estrobiome & Hormone Health

*Another part of the puzzle regarding gut
health and this relates to hormone regulation*

We have just touched on the microbiome and its importance for gut health and your immune system. This collection of microbes within your body has a far-reaching impact on your health, influencing everything from the absorption of nutrients and mood to metabolism and immunity.

Research is coming forward on specific microbes within your gut microbiome, which play a central role in the regulation of hormones - especially estrogen. This is called the **estrobolome** which influences the metabolism of various forms of estrogen and in turn the possible risk of developing estrogen-related diseases.

The Connection between Gut-Hormones and the Estrobolome

This particular group of microbes not only affect the metabolism of various forms of estrogen, they also have an effect on the balance of hormones circulating in your system, as well as the level of hormones being excreted from your body. This is obviously very relevant for those who suffer endometriosis, especially if they are estrogen dominant.

Microbes in the estrobolome produce an enzyme called beta-glucuronidase (enzymes that catalyse the breakdown of complex carbohydrates) which alters estrogens into their active forms, which can bind to estrogen receptors and influence estrogen-dependent bodily processes. The effect of having too much beta-glucuronidase in your gut is that less estrogen is excreted from the body, which means more remains within the body to be recirculated.

Balancing Your Estrobolome

The composition of your estrobolome can be influenced by many factors including diet, exposure to environmental toxins and medications. Therefore, you can support a healthy estrobolome and balance of estrogen in your body through a combination of detoxification, diet, and supplements to encourage the body to restore hormone balance. (*We look at nutrients to balance estrogen and progesterone levels further on*).

Eat a Hormone-Balancing Diet

Diet strongly influences the composition of the estrobolome. Several dietary factors may have a positive impact on the estrobolome which include:

- Probiotics strains such as Lactobacillus acidophilus can help decrease bacteria that produce beta-glucuronidase.
- Plant-based foods high in dietary fibre support healthy gut bacteria and lead to more balanced levels of estrogen.
- Cruciferous vegetables such as broccoli, cauliflower, cabbage, and kale are helpful in regulating beneficial gut bacteria, supplying fibre to keep the gut healthy and supporting healthy detoxification of hormones including estrogen.

Reduce Toxicity

Many manmade compounds called xeno-estrogens, can mimic natural estrogens in the body as well as alter the composition of the microbiome. There are several steps you can take to reduce your exposure to xeno-estrogens in everyday life by reducing your use of toiletries and household cleaning products that are full of toxic chemicals. We go into more details about reducing your toxin exposure further on in the book.

Supplements To Heal The Gut

*Here we look at the variety of supplements and nutrients
you can use to help heal your gut, some of which
are also helpful for endometriosis symptoms*

You need to be selective when using supplements, only trying one at a time to be able to assess any benefits. Follow the instructions provided with each product for dosage.

Probiotics - Supplementing with a full spectrum probiotic is a key element of **healing a damaged gut** as well as supporting friendly gut bacteria. Probiotics are also an important regime to heal the gut after taking anti-biotics.

Marshmallow root - Marshmallow root contains the amino acid proline that helps build protein in the body for tissue repair. Marshmallow root can help to heal **Leaky Gut** by creating a protective layer around the GI cell junctions. Marshmallow also soothes inflamed intestines and supports elimination of waste. You can take marshmallow root as a tea, tincture, powder or as a supplement.

Aloe vera Juice - Aloe vera is anti-inflammatory and **healing for the lining of the gut** and also acts as a prebiotic. Aloe can improve nutrient absorption and aid with better digestion overall. It also promotes a healthy balance of bacteria in the gut by supporting the growth of probiotics. Aloe is good for your health overall because it's extremely nutrient rich and contains minerals such as calcium, potassium, zinc, magnesium, manganese, and copper as well as vitamins A, B, C, and E.

Clinical studies have shown that Aloe Vera can be used to **aid the treatment of endometriosis.** As well as being rich in vitamins and minerals it is also one of the few plants that contain vitamin B12 which can increase energy. Aloe can help boost healing by 30 percent and its anti-inflammatory properties can help with the inflammation of endometriosis.

Quercetin - Quercetin is an anti-oxidant, healing herb that is shown to help heal a **leaky intestinal lining**. Quercetin prevents the release of histamine and puts a stop to allergic reactions that trigger a leaky gut reaction. Being a potent antioxidant, quercetin can also help remove damaging free radicals in the body. Additionally, **quercetin is anti-inflammatory** and may help reduce pain caused by inflammation.

Collagen - Collagen helps heal the structure and mucosal lining of your digestive tract, as we have covered earlier. Collagen is comprised of several important amino acids for gut health, including glycine which helps your body make glutathione, an important antioxidant that protects your cells. L-glutamine is another amino acid found in collagen that supports intestinal health by both **maintaining the gut barrier** and regulating metabolism.

Digestive enzymes - Digestive enzyme supplements are designed to be taken just before, or during meals to supplement the enzymes your body already produces. This will help the breakdown of your food to obtain your nutrients. Some digestive enzyme supplements contain berberine which can help to **control the over-growth caused by SIBO.** Berberine also has antioxidant, anti-inflammatory, antibacterial, and antiviral properties. (*More on digestive enzymes further on*)

N-acetyl-glucosamine – NAC - N-acetyl glucosamine really is one of the best supplements **for leaky gut.** This compound not only targets bad bacteria, but also encourages good bacteria to thrive. Glucosamine is well known for being good for bone and cartilage health, treating IBD, and can support your immune system. This nutrient also supports the growth of the gut-protective probiotic strains of Bifidobacterium. Interestingly, this supplement is reported to also help with anxiety which is probably by the action of **supporting healthy gut bacteria.**

Caprylic acid – from coconut oil - Coconut oil is very healing for the gut and has been found to reduce the over-growth of yeast in the gut. It is very easy to add coconut into your diet by adding a spoonful to your meals – great added to morning oats. The caprylic acid is also helpful in dealing with the over-growth of **SIBO.**

Probiotics For A Healthy Gut Flora

We have briefly touched on using probiotics for gut health - here we go into more detail on the benefits of these micro-organisms for your health.

The benefits of probiotics have been proven effective in supporting immune-function, reducing inflammation, promoting healthy digestion as well as absorption of nutrients. Our intestinal flora should have a natural balance of friendly bacteria which undertake a variety of vital tasks for our health. The number of bacteria in our intestines alone is much higher than the number of cells in our bodies. However, with long term use of antibiotics, drugs and hormone treatments these friendly bacteria can be destroyed.

You can replace this healthy intestinal flora by supplementing with a good quality broad-spectrum probiotic. Probiotics can also be found in certain foods such as yogurt, kefir, sauerkraut, kimchi and other fermented foods like pickles. However, many with endometriosis can have a bad reaction to some of these foods with gut distress or have a histamine reaction due to many of these foods being high in histamine.

Taking a probiotic supplement is a way around this problem, but if you have histamine intolerance and you use the wrong strain of probiotic, then this can set off a histamine reaction. You need to use a probiotic product that is made specifically for those with a histamine intolerance – more details on this further on.

Probiotics provide various health benefits

- Replacing the friendly intestinal bacteria destroyed by broad-spectrum antibiotics - these bacteria aid digestion and help suppress disease-causing bacteria
- Boost immunity and reduce inflammation
- Decrease inflammation in the gut
- Reducing the recurrence rate of lower urinary tract infections and cystitis (bladder inflammation)
- Preventing recurring vaginal infections
- Possibly enhancing immune functions in immune compromised individuals
- Aiding the production of some B vitamins and vitamin K, and aiding in the breakdown of food
- Certain strains support mental health by aiding the production of neurotransmitters and can help with anxiety and depression
- Alleviating symptoms of irritable bowel syndrome and address candida
- Protect against food allergies

The Importance Of Digestive Enzymes

Consuming good food is only part of the requirement in order to improve your health. An equally important task is actually digesting and utilizing the food you eat, and sometimes we don't always digest our foods properly due to stress and illness.

Food needs to be broken down into smaller, simpler compounds before your body can absorb them. This important process of breaking down food for its nutritional components is performed by enzymes, which are either the products of your microbiome or found naturally in your digestive tract.

However, sometimes our body's natural processes are compromised, and we need supplemental support. There are various reasons your body may need assistance from digestive enzyme supplements, such as digestive disorders, low stomach acid as well as ill-health and the stress of dealing with disease. In such cases, supporting your digestive enzymes can decrease the burden of digestion on the digestive organs and help you to absorb much needed nutrients.

Digestive enzyme supplements are available in various combinations of ingredients. The aim of these ingredients is to assist in the digestion of food and sometimes ingredients are added that help to promote your natural bile production. Some of the common ingredients include ox bile, betaine, protease, amylase, lipase and peppermint.

Interestingly, ox bile can help to treat SIBO. Bile is antimicrobial and it is the antimicrobial properties of bile that prevent bacteria from overgrowing in the small intestine which is what happens in the case of small intestinal bacterial overgrowth.

Sunflower lecithin can also be used to increase bile flow. Sunflower lecithin contains phosphatidyl-choline which helps to prevent fatty liver and helps keep bile thin and flowing easily from a sluggish gallbladder. When sufficient bile flows from the gallbladder the antimicrobial properties of bile can knock down small intestinal bacterial overgrowth and can also reduce the development of SIBO.

Supporting your digestive system by adding digestive enzymes will assist in your digestive processes and help you to get maximum nutrition from your food. Another major benefit from using digestive enzymes is that they can help to reduce the bloat, pain and discomfort caused by endo-belly. This is due to the support they provide for your digestion and can also help reduce inflammation in the gut.

Detox To Support Your Liver

You have probably read many times how important it is to look after the health of your liver and this is because the liver does so much work in detoxing your body as well as helping to clear excess estrogen from your system.

Your liver is a VITAL cleansing organ for the entire body. It cleans and filters everything that travels through your bloodstream. This includes toxins from food, skincare products, waste chemicals and by-products from drugs.

The liver also plays a vital role in flushing excess hormones from your system, as well as regulating your immune system by destroying old red and white blood cells. Consequently, your liver has a lot of work to do. When your liver is working efficiently and coping with the amount of cleansing work required, then your body will stay in balance and you will not suffer the effects of toxic overload.

This is vital for women with endometriosis, so that you can release surplus hormones and toxins, which will give the immune system the opportunity to work where it is needed – helping to tackle endometriosis.

How to jump-start your liver detox

Here is a simple liver detox program which will help to kick start your healing and improve the functions of your liver

- Drink plenty of water throughout the day to 'wash out' your system. Start the day with some lemon water to promote your digestive process
- No sugar, alcohol, caffeine, gluten – these foods are advised to omit from the diet to help endometriosis, so you will be on to a good start
- Begin the first 2 days with very clean and simple meals like salads, vegetable soups or stir fry veg – this period allows your body to adjust in readiness for the next couple of days
- After 2 days simplify the diet further for another 2 days to 'deepen' the detox – juices, raw foods like salads, steamed veg, baked veg, and herb teas
- Then for days 5 to 14 introduce whole-grains and simple protein like organic chicken and fish.
- Get plenty of rest, some fresh air, and gentle exercise like walking during this period

Do not use chemical-based toiletries as these chemicals will be absorbed through your skin and will undermine the detox process.

You may feel sluggish and tired to start with as the toxins are off-loaded, but as the days go by you should hopefully feel more energy.

If you continue with this simple diet regime for about a month before adding other foods to your diet, you should start to feel more energised, improve your immune system, along with supporting the health of your liver; your body will then be able to really focus on dealing with endometriosis.

We look at the Elimination diet further on, which will help you get to the root of your specific food intolerances. However, doing a liver detox is something you can do to give your system a clean-out, especially if you have been taking any drugs treatments, for example you have been on a course of anti-biotics, or you have recently had surgery and want to flush out the anaesthetics and pain meds from your system. However, do not do a detox immediately after surgery, you need time for your body to recover first. Allow yourself at least three weeks before undertaking a detox.

Foods that will support your liver

Garlic - This pungent white bulb has the ability to activate liver enzymes that help your body flush out toxins. Garlic also holds high amounts of allicin and selenium, two natural compounds that aid in liver cleansing.

Grapefruit - High in vitamin C and antioxidants, grapefruit increases the natural cleansing processes of the liver. A small glass of freshly-squeezed grapefruit juice will help boost production of liver detoxification enzymes that help flush out toxins

Beets and carrots - Both extremely high in plant-flavonoids and beta-carotene, eating both beets and carrots can help stimulate and improve overall liver function. Beets are also good for getting a boost in iron.

Leafy green vegetables - One of the best foods for cleansing the liver, leafy greens can be eaten raw, cooked or juiced. Greens literally soak up environmental toxins from the blood stream. They also have the ability to neutralize heavy metals, chemicals and pesticides.

Apples - Apples contain malic acid which supports the liver and gallbladder. They are also high in pectin which helps the body to releases toxins.

Oils - Cold-pressed organic oils such as olive, and hemp are great for the liver, when used in moderation. They help the body by providing a lipid base that can suck up harmful toxins in the body.

Lemons and limes - These citrus fruits contain very high amounts of the vitamin C, which aids the body in synthesising toxins into a substance that can be absorbed by water. Drinking freshly-squeezed lemon or lime juice in the morning helps stimulate the liver as well as your digestive system.

Whole grains - Grains, such as brown rice, are rich in B-complex vitamins, nutrients known to improve overall fat metabolism, liver function and liver decongestion

Supporting the liver with supplements

*The following is a list of vitamins and supplements
known to be supportive for liver health.*

Alpha-lipoic acid - A primary function of ALA is to increase the body's production of glutathione, which helps dissolve toxic substances in the liver. ALA can also help with nerve pain. ALA also support mitochondria function which aids in energy production.

Artichoke - It contains cynarine, a substance that aids the liver in boosting the production of bile that helps speed up the movement of food and waste. This makes detoxification processes in the body more efficient, helping various organs to clear out harmful toxins such as alcohol and other chemicals. Artichoke is a common ingredient in many liver support supplement blends.

Choline - A macronutrient present in the form of phosphatidylcholine, choline is a compound that makes up the structural component of fat. Choline is particularly important for liver health as it is required for the proper transportation of fat from the liver to cells throughout the body. Another of the major benefits of choline is its role in keeping the liver free from harmful toxic build-up.

Dandelion root - Its natural diuretic properties enhance the liver's ability to efficiently rid the body of toxins, thus strengthening the immune system and alleviating indigestion, among other benefits.

NAC (N-acetyl-cysteine) - we have already looked at this supplement to help heal the gut. NAC is a potent antioxidant and a precursor to glutathione and has been shown to heal the liver and can prevent liver damage from drug use. During detoxification, NAC is essential for replenishing and maintaining glutathione levels in the body. The most important quality of NAC for women with endometriosis is that research shows that NAC effectively treats ovarian endometriosis, it can **help in the reduction in cyst sizes** and has no side effects.

Milk thistle - Perhaps the most often mentioned compound when it comes to supporting liver health. Milk Thistle also repairs damage to the liver cells caused by disease, alcohol, and drugs. Silymarin works by acting like a gatekeeper, protecting the liver from toxins and free radicals. Milk thistle also helps to prevent the depletion of glutathione. The antioxidant activity of this important compound is believed to be ten times more potent than Vitamin E.

I have noted there is confusion in the endometriosis community as to whether Milk Thistle is estrogenic. It is the leaves and flowers of Milk Thistle that are estrogenic, but the seeds are not estrogenic. When looking for a supplement of Milk Thistle ensure it is derived from the seeds.

This is a supplement that deserves to be included in your treatment schedule as it has many benefits which include:

- Milk Thistle can reduce estrogen by speeding its clearance from the body.

- The active ingredient in milk thistle, silymarin, acts as an antioxidant by reducing free radical production.
- Milk Thistle stimulates bile production within the liver. Bile production is really important to help break down fats in the body and absorb nutrients.
- It repairs the cells found in the liver which means it has the ability to physically repair the liver.
- It reduces the formation of the negative prostaglandins that cause inflammation and reduces the auto-immune reaction in some patients.

Be careful not to take Milk Thistle close to meals as it can reduce absorption of iron

Diet &

Nutrition

for

Endometriosis

'The food you eat can be either the safest and most powerful form of medicine or the slowest form of poison.'

Ann Wigmore

Feedback following diet changes...

'After being on the endometriosis diet for the last couple of months I thought I would drop you a line and tell you how things have been going.

I was a bit put out at the thought of cutting so many things from my diet, but if you want to give yourself the best outcome you just have to bite the bullet and do it. I have been pretty diligent and could not believe the difference in how I have felt, not only in regards to when I have my period but also the rest of the time.

I don't feel "weighed down" and sluggish, and have a lot more energy throughout the day. And this just from changing your diet. Even people I have told about this who do not suffer from endometriosis cannot believe how very much of a difference can be had from changing your diet. I feel so much better and have had just 2 periods since beginning the diet.

With each one the pain has got less and my periods have been lighter. I have only had to take painkillers one time, and only on one day. I can only hope things keep diminishing the longer I am on this diet. And I really don't feel like calling it a diet. It is a way of life now. I am even starting to adjust recipes!!!

I was always more into the natural side of things. I thank you for doing all the hard yards on behalf of so many of us sufferers.'

Staying in good health – Ariana

‹I purchased a copy of the book some time ago and have found it invaluable. I kept meaning to write and say thank you. Cutting wheat, dairy, and sugar out of my diet (about 80% of the time is all I can manage) has made a huge difference to my well-being already. My partner eats whatever I cook and he says that your recipes are the best vegetarian recipes he has ever had! He loves our new diet!

I am more than happy for you to use my e-mail as a testimony. You might also like to add that as well as the new diet alleviating my stomach cramps and pain, I lost weight, stopped bloating, and my lower back symptoms disappeared (provided I stick to no meat/dairy/wheat/sugar of course)!'

Rochelle, Australia

'I was told of your web site by a co-worker and thought the diet couldn't hurt. Within two cycles, my symptoms disappeared. It totally made sense that everything I was eating before had so much outside hormones, it couldn't possibly help regulate my own hormones. By following this diet, I became a healthier person overall, I wasn't tired as much, I had more energy, just felt better.

In 2016 I gave birth to a healthy little boy and something my previous doctors told me was not likely. There were no complications whatsoever, he is an absolute blessing. Thank you, thank you, thank you for all of your research on this disease and sharing what you've learned. God Bless You'
Christine

On average, U.S. medical schools offer only 19.6 hours of nutrition education across four years of medical school, according to a 2010 report in Academic Medicine.

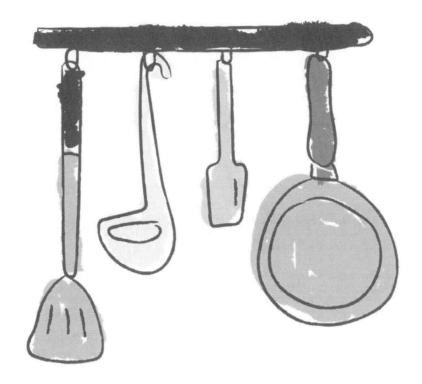

where the magic
happens!!

You Need The Right Diet For You

Once upon a time using diet to help endometriosis wasn't even on the radar. You can now find many websites, numerous articles, books and even support groups which focus on diet and endometriosis.

As a nutritionist who specializes in endometriosis, I have found that there are many variations to using diet for endometriosis. My research and my experience have shown me that each woman is individual and there is no cookie-cutter diet.

Some of the advice you may have found regarding diet for endometriosis can seem overwhelming, confusing and even contradictory, especially when certain individuals provide advice which may be based on limited knowledge or personal experience. Using diet is *very individual* and what may work for one may not work for another – how often have you heard that phrase?

It was the use of good nutrition that helped me on my own road to recovery as you have read in my story. Food is your fuel. It's what runs your engine and nourishes your entire body. The foods you eat can really influence your mood and your emotions as well as your energy levels.

The cells in your body are ALL replaced over time, even your bones and your liver — your whole body becomes replaced. So, what you eat today will influence how your body is rebuilt in the future.

When you follow an anti-inflammatory diet and leave out foods that can trigger your endometriosis symptoms you will gradually feel the benefits. Many women say it takes them around 3 to 4 weeks before they feel improvements with less symptoms.

But when you slip up and go back to old habits and eat the wrong foods you will soon feel it - it usually triggers a nasty flare with pain and bloating. This is something I found out myself – my biggest problem foods were gluten and coffee, and if I had any carbonated drinks I would be in agony for hours.

When you eat the right foods with a nourishing healing diet, you can reduce the amount of estrogens in your system, reduce your inflammation, reduce your toxic load as well as improve your immune system. All these benefits will help to reduce your symptoms. We look at how you can find the right diet for you next.

Elimination Diet

Discover your particular food triggers

Undertaking an elimination diet can be an important starting point to help you discover your particular food intolerances, which in turn will help to heal the gut as well as improve many symptoms of endometriosis.

The principle to an elimination diet is to stop eating certain foods that are known to cause digestive and health problems, and to pinpoint which are your particular trigger foods. You then gradually re-introduce foods one at a time to see how your body reacts.

It is advised not to cut out everything all at once when doing and elimination diet, as it is safer and easier to do this in stages, otherwise you may go through a rough detox process. Choose one item or food group per week to eliminate until you have reached the goal of eliminating all foods that are part of the elimination diet protocol.

The key foods that are removed for an elimination diet include:

- Gluten
- Dairy
- Soy
- Sugar
- Corn
- Peanuts
- Shellfish
- Processed foods
- Eggs
- Citrus
- Alcohol
- Processed meats and red meat
- Nightshades – tomatoes, peppers, eggplant, potatoes and onions

The time-frame to do an elimination diet is about ten weeks and this includes the time to eliminate various food groups as well as an adjustment period. But it may take longer – there is no rush and you can take it at your own pace. It takes time for your body to flush the trigger foods from your system, and even longer for your body to stop reacting and your symptoms to clear.

Additional benefits - it has been found that doing an elimination diet can help to get to the root of Irritable Bowel Syndrome as well as Leaky Gut.

Foods suggestions to eat on an elimination diet include:

- Oily fish like salmon and mackerel – aim for wild caught fish
- Organic chicken
- Eat lots of fibre, especially fresh veggies
- Fruits except citrus
- Grains including rice and quinoa
- Eat lots of healthy fats like coconut oil, walnut oil and avocados

This is a restrictive diet and should only be done for as long as it takes to go through the process. Some will advise to eliminate all meat for an elimination diet, but I feel as long as you eat organic chicken or wild caught fish then eating animal protein will be OK.

Reintroducing foods

After the allotted time, you then choose to eat one of the foods you have eliminated, like dairy or eggs. You then monitor to see how you feel over the next 48 hours. If you have no reaction after two days then try the same food again for a second time and notice how you feel.

If you still have no reaction, you can then re-introduce this food into your diet. You follow these same steps for each food group, being sure to take notes to monitor how you feel.

Some meal ideas when doing an elimination diet:

- Oatmeal with coconut or almond milk for breakfast
- Green smoothies for breakfast
- Chia pudding made with coconut milk
- Large green salads sprinkled with sesame seeds of chia seeds, sliced avocado
- Roasted sweet potatoes with roasted root veggies
- Simple grilled fish with salad
- Simple light veggie soups
- Sprouted seeds/bean salad mix
- Simple veggies, stews, casseroles
- Fruits – those not on the FODMAP list - *below*
- Nuts or roast kale chips for snacking

Ensure to eat fats to help support stable blood sugar levels – put a spoonful of coconut oil in your green smoothies or chia pudding.

Make sure you are getting sufficient nutrients, and eating sprouted seeds and grains will provide you with plenty of nutrients. Also, chia and hemp seeds will also provide you with great nutrients.

Drink plenty of water, as doing an elimination diet can be like doing a detox, which will off-load toxins from your system and water will help to flush out these toxins.

So principally an elimination diet is done in two phases – eliminate major food groups as mentioned and then gradually re-introduce foods, monitoring how your body reacts.

FODMAP DIET – a specific elimination diet

FODMAP is an acronym for "Fermentable Oligo-, Di-, Mono-saccharides And Polyols". They are short chain carbohydrates that are poorly absorbed in the small intestine.

The specific diet regime known as the FODMAP diet eliminates certain short chain carbohydrates, specifically – gluten, lactose, and fructose. These food groups tend to ferment in the gut and can cause abdominal pain, bloating and diarrhoea or constipation. The principle of the FODMAP diet is similar to the elimination diet, but focussed on specific food groups as mentioned.

The FODMAP diet also includes an elimination phase, lasting anything from 3 to 8 weeks. Once again, stage two involves reintroducing foods one at a time to identify which foods are causing an intolerance. At this stage you test specific foods for two to three days with each food.

FODMAP foods you remove include:

Dairy: cream cheese, milk, yoghurt, cream

Vegetables: garlic, onions, asparagus, brussel sprouts, cauliflower, artichoke. leeks, mushrooms, tomato paste

Grains: wheat, amaranth, barley, rye, soybean products

Pulses: black-eye peas, broad beans, butter beans, chickpeas, kidney beans, lentils, soy beans, split peas

Fruit: apples, apricots, blackberries, cherries, currants, mangoes, nectarines, peaches, pears, plumbs, watermelon, dried fruit

Safe foods for the FODMAP diet

Vegetables: courgettes, peas, green beans, carrots, sweet potatoes, avocado, squash, beets, lettuce, celery, cucumber, parsnip, spinach, olives, bell peppers, cabbage, green beans,

Fruit: blueberries, kiwi, pineapple, rhubarb, strawberries, papaya, banana, grapes, raspberries

Carbs: rice, quinoa, rice noodles, oats, gluten free pasta, lentils

Protein: all animal protein is seen as safe for the FODMAP diet but ideally needs to be organic and free of chemicals. Also processed and cured meats would need to be removed.

Endometriosis, Histamine & Diet

As we know endometriosis often means being estrogen dominant, and estrogen may play a role in the development of histamine intolerance. How does this happen? ... well, the more estrogen that is circulating in your body the more histamine will be released. At the same time, histamine stimulates estrogen, leading to a vicious circle. (*Oh great, I hear you say! Don't worry, this is manageable*)

This problem is usually worse just before menstruation and during ovulation. This is when estrogen is higher that progesterone, so in turn your body makes even more histamine. Additionally, tissue in the cells of connective tissue close to damaged sites such as adhesions and endometrial implants release histamine in reaction to the damage.

Histamine is a naturally occurring compound that helps regulate specific functions of your digestive, nervous, and immune system. Your body normally regulates histamine, first by producing histamine and then by clearing it with the enzymes histamine N-methyltransferase (HNMT) and diamine oxidase (DAO).

When your DAO levels are too low, it's difficult for your body to efficiently metabolize and excrete excess histamine. As a result, histamine levels rise, leading to various physical symptoms. Common symptoms of a histamine reaction include itchy skin, sneezing, face flushing, headaches, dry mouth, nasal congestion, high heart rate and can also include anxiety as well as irregular menstrual cycles.

Various factors may contribute to diminished DAO activity or overproduction of histamine, including alcohol use, certain medications, intestinal bacterial overgrowth, and eating large amounts of histamine-containing foods.

Taking pain medication, antibiotics and muscle relaxants can also interfere with the enzyme DOA, which can then cause an imbalance of histamines in the body. You have probably taken many pain meds over time, so this can set you up for developing histamine problems. Other factors that can interfere with DOA activity includes stress, injury and intestinal conditions including damage to the gut lining – all of these seem to be familiar for those with endometriosis.

Histamine Elimination Diet

It can be helpful to eliminate high histamine foods for a while, as this will assess whether you do have a histamine issue caused by these foods. This is similar to the Elimination Diet and you will be removing foods that are known to be high in histamines, and then reintroduce foods one by one and assess for a negative reaction.

High histamine foods include:

- fermented dairy products, such as cheese (especially aged), yogurt, sour cream, buttermilk, and kefir
- fermented vegetables, such as sauerkraut and kimchi
- pickles or pickled veggies
- kombucha
- cured or fermented meats, such as sausages, salami, and fermented ham
- all alcoholic drinks
- fermented soy products such as tempeh, miso, soy sauce, and natto
- fermented grains, such as sourdough bread
- frozen or canned fish such as sardines and tuna
- eggplant
- spinach
- tomatoes
- vinegar
- tomato ketchup
- peas
- mushrooms

It's difficult to quantify the exact amount of histamine in food – which is why you'll find contradicting information and several different food lists on the internet.

How to manage histamine issues

Certain supplements can help you manage histamine intolerance

- Supplement with vitamin B6 as it upregulates DAO.
- DAO is also found as a supplement that is frequently used to treat histamine intolerance. DAO supplements work to break down histamine from diet sources
- Supplement with quercetin as it is known to help reduce histamine levels.

- Supplement with bromelain, which is a compound found in high concentration in the stem of pineapples and has been found to be effective in treating histamine issues. Bromelain can also help reduce inflammation, especially in the gut and can help reduce pain and inflammation of endometriosis.
- Vitamin C can help reduce histamine release and make histamine break down faster once it is released.

Histamines and probiotic products

If you have a histamine problem you need to take care which probiotic product you use as certain strains can increase histamines, therefore making your histamine problem even worse.

When shopping for a probiotic complex look for a product that states it is safe to take for those with histamine issues. One such product is ProBiota HistaminX from Seeking Health. Another product that is suitable is Flora Symmetry from Vitanica.

Testing For Intolerances

There are different commercial tests you can use to test for food intolerances which include blood tests, hair analysis tests and finger-prick blood test to check for IgE or IgG-4 antibodies to certain foods. It is questionable as to whether these tests are always accurate or reliable, and often private laboratories may be simply cashing in on the health market.

For example, your IgG antibody levels will fluctuate daily depending on what you have been eating recently. The advice from experts is that IgG tests should not be used as an attempt to diagnose any food intolerances. Medical advice is that doing an elimination diet is the best 'test' to find out if you have any food intolerances.

I recently watched a TV program where the presenter, who is a doctor, sent off a blood test and hair test to check for food intolerances. They were sent to two separate laboratories and the results came back with some totally contradictory results. So, it seems you cannot rely on these types of food intolerance tests, but using a reliable laboratory you may be able to obtain a decent bench-mark.

Histamine Intolerance test

Testing for histamine intolerance can include a blood test to check for DAO levels and enzyme activity levels. Another way to diagnose histamine intolerance is with a prick test, where a histamine solution is applied which tests for a reaction to the solution. Also, an allergist can test for food allergies and food intolerances to assess for histamine intolerance.

Should you have tests for intolerances and gut problems?

This question is very much individual and may depend how severe your gut symptoms are and you are noticing a definite link between what you eat and the severity of your symptoms. Your physician may be willing to order these tests, but if they won't order tests then you are reliant on the cost of private testing.

As I have just mentioned, the efficacy of certain tests can be questionable and you may not obtain accurate results, particularly for food intolerance tests and sometimes SIBO tests may be inaccurate.

Your best option is to do an elimination diet, to include removing high histamine foods. This gives you much better control, will save you money on any testing, and the results will be very specific to you.

Food intolerances, histamine intolerance, Leaky gut and Candida can often be assessed and managed through diet, and adding in specific digestive support supplements. These include digestive enzymes, probiotics and gut healing nutrients like collagen, colostrum, and aloe vera juice can all go a long way to healing your gut.

SIBO is the difficult one, and you may need medical guidance to help with diagnosis and treatment especially as SIBO can lead to nutrient deficiencies.

—————～—————

Putting This Altogether

We have covered a number of topics related to gut health, the microbiome, detox and specific diets, but how do you put this altogether and put this into action.

The Elimination Diet – This is a good place to start and will help to get to the root cause of some of your symptoms and find your trigger foods. Women I have worked with have found the exercise of doing the elimination diet to be extremely useful and takes out the guess work.

FODMAP diet - to discover if you have problems with FODMAP foods you need to remove the foods as listed, and then reintroduce these foods to assess for any reactions, which is a similar process to the Elimination diet.

Histamine Elimination Diet - It has been found that endometrial implants release histamine due to the inflammatory response, so regulating histamine release will help to reduce the histamine response. The most common foods that are triggers for histamine release are mostly fermented foods including fermented soy products plus a few specific vegetables. These should not prove difficult to remove from your diet, and to help control a histamine reaction you can use specific supplements as mentioned earlier.

Combining diets – You have the option to combine the Elimination/FODMAP diets, and you will get your answers quicker, rather than trying to do separate elimination diets. You will still have sufficient food choices to be able to provide a nutritious diet for the time of going through this process. However, this needs to be done slowly, there is no rush, and you need to be prepared by gathering healthy recipe ideas and ensure you are covering your nutritional needs.

Alternatively, you could undertake separate elimination diets if you feel doing them together is too stressful. However, many foods cross-over and are included on the list of foods to remove for both the Elimination and FODMAP diet, so you only have to remove a few more foods.

This may seem like a lot of hard work and you may feel you suffer enough hardship because of endometriosis, but you only have to do this once. The time and effort will be worth it and will highlight which foods to omit so that you can eat a diet that does not cause gut distress, bloating and increased pain. The end result will be worth it and will pay dividends.

Monitoring symptoms

When I suffered endometriosis, as well as monitoring particular food reactions, I also had to uncover other very specific dietary triggers. For example, I had to monitor which foods I could safely combine together without causing problems, what I could safely eat on an empty stomach, and even the time of day could affect how my digestive system worked and whether I would end up with bloating and the infamous endo-belly.

This is why keeping a food journal is so important so that you can take note of your triggers. Additionally, your symptoms can have other triggers such as stress, lack of sleep, or not eating enough causing you to have unstable blood-sugar levels. Take note of all these issues – monitoring all your symptoms is going to help you get to the bottom of the causes of your symptom triggers.

Tips to prepare for an Elimination Diet

- Write down a list of all the food groups you need to remove from your diet and start making a food and symptoms diary.
- Before you start, ensure you have plenty of simple and clean recipe ideas to make the process less stressful – lots of nourishing salads, plenty of veggie dishes, veggie soups, fresh fruit, herbs teas, green tea.
- Check out blog pages and websites that have advice about the elimination diet and FODMAP diet and check for recipe and snack ideas to help reduce the anxiety of knowing what to eat.
- Ensure you are covering your nutritional needs which can include foods like sprouted grains, seeds and nuts. Also make sure you have sufficient protein which can include chicken, turkey and fish – ensure you eat organic white meat and wild caught fish.
- Aim to eat three meals a day and have a snack in between to help control blood sugar levels.
- Start to remove food groups one at a time and allow a time gap of around a week between each diet change.
- Remember to keep up with your diary of your progress and when you start to add foods back in - this is when your diary becomes even more important.
- Take this slowly and don't rush through an elimination diet. You do not want to be going through a heavy-duty detox (however you may still go through a detox process by default – which is no bad thing). Ensure to drink plenty of water to help flush the toxins being released as your diet becomes cleaner.
- Try to keep your pain medication to a minimum and use natural alternatives instead
- Use additional detox tools to help ease the process including Epsom salts baths, skin brushing and castor oil packs (*details further in the book*)

The Elimination Process

Step 1: Eliminating gluten which includes bread, cookies, pastries etc. You can use rice and quinoa to provide some carbs in your diet. Stop all processed foods

Step 2: Remove all sugars and only use natural alternatives of honey or stevia

Step 3: Cut out all soy products. You can use coconut aminos instead of soy sauce

Step 4: Remove all dairy including milk – you can use oat, coconut or rice milk instead. Ensure to eat plenty of dark leafy green veggies to provide calcium and chia seeds and sesame seeds will also provide calcium

Step 5: Remove red meat and any processed meat products, cured meats and shell-fish. For protein you can eat organic free-range chicken and oily fish like salmon and trout

Step 6: Remove histamine foods and nightshades – peas, mushrooms, peppers, tomatoes and fermented and pickled foods, maybe removing fermented and pickled foods first, then move onto the other foods rather than removing these foods all in one go

Allow a week for each step of the elimination process, plus allow a few more weeks for your system to 'settle'. Use this time to closely monitor your symptoms. By the time you have eliminated all food groups you should start to feel the difference.

It is then time to start adding in food groups one at a time and take note of any reaction or changes in symptoms. Go through this process with each food group allowing at least a week for each new food group being added back in. This gives you time to really listen to your body.

Once you have gone through the elimination diet you should have learnt what your trigger foods are and be able to take action and adjust your diet.

Putting this into action regards endometriosis

Many of the foods you will be testing with the elimination diets are similar to the diet guidelines to help reduce the symptoms of endometriosis. If you do not have a reaction to certain foods then you know you can keep these in your diet without causing problems.

We look next at the dietary recommendations for endometriosis. This advice is based on reliable research, nutritional common-sense, backed up by experiences of endometriosis sufferers who have had success using diet changes to improve their symptoms.

I have read a few contradictions to this advice, some of which are quite misleading including advice from various sources in the endometriosis community advising that soy is OK to eat, which is far from the truth – soy is one of the most intensely sprayed crops as well as being a genetically modified crop, not to mention that it is very high in phyto-estrogens.

I have also read an endometriosis health blog saying that gluten it totally safe to eat with endometriosis – this is really bad advice, and there are a number of research articles that indicate the benefits of a gluten free diet for endometriosis which is consistently endorsed by endometriosis sufferers. This is even more relevant with auto-immune diseases, as gluten can cause real problems for those with auto-immune issues.

We are all different, and react differently to certain foods, but to make sweeping statements saying certain foods are totally safe (which some have found to cause bad symptoms of pain and bloating) is very bad advice.

I repeat, that if you learn for yourself which foods cause a problem for you having gone through the elimination diet, then you are on to a good footing and you will then know what you can and cannot eat – all common sense, and individual to you.

cooking is love

Aim Of Diet To Reduce Your Symptoms

Making diet changes to help endometriosis is a multi-faceted regime – diet can help with symptoms by reducing pain and inflammation, balance hormones, heal the gut, support stable blood sugar levels to help sustain energy, support the immune system and help reduce further development of endometriosis.

Reduce inflammation

Endometriosis causes inflammation especially where there is damage caused by cysts and adhesions. Inflammation can also occur in the digestive tract which can be caused when endometriosis infiltrates the digestive tract, especially the bowel. Changing your diet to an anti-inflammatory diet will help to reduce inflammation and in turn will help reduce pain.

Balance hormones

When dealing with endometriosis you need to keep estrogen levels under control as estrogen feeds the development of endometriosis. Certain foods contain phyto-estrogens, however they are not as potent as the bodies own estrogens. Eating some phyto-estrogenic foods can help to block estrogen receptors which will reduce the effect of your own estrogen hormones.

Reducing pain

Certain foods can cause pain and inflammation as they increase negative prostaglandins that are responsible for causing pain and inflammation in the body. By reducing your intake of foods that increase prostaglandins you will obviously be able to reduce pain and inflammation.

Gut health

Gut inflammation, leaky gut, and SIBO can contribute to poor absorption of nutrients which can result in poor immune health and inflammation. Eating foods that support the gut and avoiding foods that irritate the gut will aid in the whole healing process. You could be eating the best diet to help endometriosis, and using anti-inflammatory herbs and spices, but if your gut health is poor, the likelihood that you are absorbing your nutrients is reduced.

Blood sugar balance

Blood sugar imbalances can lead to inflammation, immune flares, hormonal imbalances, and compromised brain function. Supporting balanced blood sugar is critical for recovery from any inflammatory condition and ensures much needed energy levels are sustained in order to reduce further stress on the body.

Nutrient density

Every system in the body needs a wide array of nutrients to function at its best, including the immune system, your reproductive system and even your brain. Nutrient-dense foods are central to the diet, giving your body the tools it needs to heal deficiencies and support every function of the body.

Reduce toxins

By eating a clean, nourishing diet and not eating toxic foods that contain chemicals, e-numbers, preservatives and pesticides will help to detox and reduce stress on the body. This will help to speed the healing process.

Immune system support

Inflammation, leaky gut, hormone imbalances, blood sugar imbalances, and micronutrient deficiencies can all contribute to a compromised immune system. By reducing bacterial overgrowth and inflammation in the gut and supporting blood sugar regulation, the diet will help to support healthy immune function. Also, there is the need to calm an over-active immune system response by avoiding certain proteins like gluten and dairy, as these can disrupt the immune-system.

Guidelines To Diet For Endometriosis

We now go into the nitty-gritty regarding diet changes to help reduce the pain and symptoms of endometriosis. Diet changes can support healing on many levels.

The new 'buzz phrase' regarding diet and endometriosis is 'There is no such thing as an endometriosis diet', which is true to some extent, as there is no hard and fast diet to help manage endometriosis. However, many have found that by following similar guidelines as outlined here, they are able to obtain a noticeable reduction of their symptoms, as well as an improvement in their overall health.

One key aim of diet to help endometriosis is to reduce inflammation. However, it goes deeper than just dealing with inflammation. You also need to ensure you are <u>not</u> eating foods that increase pain through particular chemical pathways.

Prostaglandins Pain And Diet

Let's look deeper at how we feel pain caused by food choices – I have gone into detail with this topic to help you get to grips with the importance of how certain foods can affect pain.

Our bodies experience pain through messenger hormones travelling through the body and they end up passing these messages to the brain. Our brains then register this message as a 'pain' response and we then feel that pain. This pain response alerts the body to a threat – like a cut, being injured, suffering inflammation within the body etc.

If you cut off these messenger hormones your brain will not register this pain. These hormones are called prostaglandins and they are found throughout your body. There are two types of prostaglandins in the body – 'good prostaglandins' and 'bad prostaglandins.' The bad ones are called Antagonistic Prostaglandins and they cause pain, inflammation, fever and blood clotting.

By making changes in your diet, you can shift the prostaglandin production from the negative inflammatory prostaglandins to the anti-inflammatory prostaglandins.

Functions of Prostaglandins - some basics

Prostaglandins have a variety of physiological effects on the body including:

- Activation of the inflammatory responses at the sites of damaged tissue, and production of pain and fever. When tissues are damaged, white blood cells flood the site to try to minimise tissue destruction. Prostaglandins are produced as a result.
- Prostaglandins assist the transmission of pain signals to the brain so that you are readily alerted that damage or dysfunction has occurred within the body.
- Blood clots form when a blood vessel is damaged. A type of prostaglandin called thromboxane stimulates constriction and clotting of platelets. Also, the opposite happens and prostaglandin 12 (PG12) is produced on the walls of blood vessels where clots should not be forming. (The body is very, very clever. It knows what to do, where to do it and when.)
- Certain prostaglandins are involved with the introduction of labour and other reproductive processes, and the role of fertility. PGE2 causes uterine contractions and has been used to induce labour.

- They are involved in several other organs and systems such as the gastrointestinal tract, cell growth and the immune system response.

Prostaglandins, womb contractions and period pain

Primary dysmenorrhoea (painful periods) is caused by cramping in the uterine muscles — the uterus is a muscle and like all muscles it contracts and relaxes! Women don't usually feel these muscles contract, unless it is a particularly strong contraction.

With endometriosis the pain associated with menstrual cramps is usually very intense and painful. During a contraction, blood supply to the uterus can be temporarily cut off. This deprives the muscle of oxygen, which causes pain. But why do the uterine muscles contract?

It is caused by the series two prostaglandins (PGE2). Series two prostaglandins help the uterus to shed the womb lining during menstruation by causing the contraction of the uterine muscles. Understandably, if too many of these prostaglandins are produced, then the contractions will be more severe and cause painful menstrual cramps — primary dysmenorrhoea.

However, not all prostaglandins have this effect on the involuntary uterine muscles, which is why diet can play a big role in minimising the production of series two prostaglandins. The types of fatty acids included in your diet influence the types of prostaglandins that are made.

For example, series two prostaglandin (the type that trigger powerful contractions of the uterus) levels are increased when animal fat is included in the diet. In contrast, series one and series three prostaglandins (the type that don't cause uterine contractions) are produced when the diet is higher in alpha-linoleic acid (omega 3).

Endometriosis, estrogen, prostaglandins and the immune-system

Endometriosis produces its own estrogen - which is why it's termed an estrogen-sensitive condition or an estrogen-dominant condition.

But what causes endometriosis to produce its own estrogen? It is caused by the immune-system and here is the process …..

Inflammatory mediators produced by the immune system are responsible and one in particular, called prostaglandin two (PGE2) activates an enzyme in the endometriosis lesion called aromatase. This enzyme is what stimulates the production of estrogen. When that estrogen is produced, it stimulates more production of PGE2. This then becomes a never-ending vicious cycle.

This is why we need to reduce your production of these negative prostaglandins and inflammation through diet, and by supporting your immune system.

Prostaglandins and Diet

The KEY way to shift the production of prostaglandins from the negative (inflammatory / pain messenger / womb contracting type) to the positive (anti-inflammatory / suppression of pain messenger type), is through your diet, and most crucially by the types of fats and oils you include in your diet.

Several enzymes take part in the process that transforms fats into prostaglandins. These enzymes act as gatekeepers, channelling fats into the making of different prostaglandins. Like other enzymes in the body, they require specific nutrient co-enzymes and nutrients to do their job especially the B vitamins.

Foods to avoid to lower prostaglandins include:

Cheeses, butter, bacon, fried meats, fast foods, beef, milk, eggs, sweet baked goods, white bread, biscuits, white rice, sweetened breakfast cereals, salad dressings, vegetable oils, corn oil, safflower oil, soy oil, peanut oil, alcohol, sugary soda, coffee.

Bromelain and prostaglandins

The enzyme bromelain from the stem of the pineapple, is also effective at inhibiting the inflammatory prostaglandins. In an extensive five-year study of more than 200 people experiencing inflammation as a result of surgery, traumatic injuries and wounds, 75 percent of the study participants had excellent improvement with bromelain. You can find bromelain as a supplement used to aid digestion, and sometimes comes blended with other ingredients as a digestive supplement.

Other foods that can reduce negative prostaglandins

Turmeric, mangosteen, and pomegranate have also shown prostaglandin-suppressing qualities, and as we know turmeric has great anti-inflammatory and pain relief benefits. According to studies green tea can help to reduce negative prostaglandins in the body, as well as other health benefits. Ginger is another food that can help reduce prostaglandins, caused by the active chemicals in ginger — gingerols and shogaols — which mediate the levels of prostaglandins. Ginger is really easy to make into a tea, which is also really good at helping nausea and upset stomach.

Best foods to increase the good prostaglandins

The best foods to promote the good prostaglandins are the foods that have high levels of omega 3 which includes oily fish like salmon, trout and mackerel. Nuts and seeds are also good sources especially chia seeds and hemp seeds.

Summary to prostaglandins

*There are 2 groups of prostaglandins
which are most relevant to endometriosis
- Good or Bad*

Good - take part in the normal functions of the body without contributing to the processes which cause the negative effects of endometriosis. Good prostaglandins have anti-inflammatory properties, i.e., they reduce pain, swelling and redness.

Bad - take part in the functions of the body which contribute to endometriosis symptoms and its negative effects i.e., pain, inflammation, digestive disturbance, connective tissue damage.

Once the bad prostaglandins have done their work with regard to injury and damage, the body then creates fibrin, which is what makes up scar tissue, to surround the injured area with a mesh-like coating. (We cover fibrin in more detail in the topic of serrapeptase).

The way your body produces different types of prostaglandins can be controlled by what you include in your diet by consumption of different oils and foods. Some foods and oils will promote the negative prostaglandins because of subtle chemical reactions. In turn, other foods and good oils will block that chemical reaction and stop the negative prostaglandins from being produced.

To conclude

Our bodies will produce prostaglandins to act as warning signals, or to provide support to damaged tissue. The dual roles of prostaglandins seem to be contradictory, but we obviously need both types of prostaglandins for the repair, maintenance and survival of the body.

If we did not suffer pain then we would not be alerted to the problem of damage within the body. Suffering pain is distressing, but in turn it is also telling us that something is wrong.

It is fortunate that we now know how these particular prostaglandins work (be it in simple terms), so that women with endometriosis are able to alter the balance of prostaglandin production to reduce their symptoms by reducing the negative prostaglandins, and aim to increase the positive prostaglandins.

Foods Advised To Remove

This is the list of foods that are advised to be removed from your diet to help reduce your symptoms and why they may cause problems

I have been as detailed as possible with this list to cover all bases, describing why certain foods are advised to be avoided. However, I will repeat, if you have undertaken an elimination diet and found you are not being affected by some of these foods, then you will know you are safe to eat them without causing problems for <u>you</u>.

Wheat - this includes breads, cakes and pasta products, all based on wheat - contains phytic acid which can aggravate symptoms of endometriosis, and can also cause inflammation. Also contain gluten which can cause inflammation and aggravate symptoms.

Gluten - Many with endometriosis seem to have a negative reaction to gluten. A 2012 study looking at endometriosis and the gluten link found that of 207 participants, 156 reported significant decrease in pain and bloating when stopping gluten. Many with endometriosis have a predisposition for additional immune-system disorders which can include hypothyroidism, and gluten can set off a thyroid auto-immune reaction. Gluten suppresses the immune system and is irritating to the intestines, which makes it harder to absorb nutrients from food.

Red meats - promotes negative prostaglandins which cause inflammation and pain and can also contain growth hormones. A 2018 study published in the American Journal of Obstetrics & Gynaecology found that a higher intake of red meat increases the risk of endometriosis by 56%.

Refined and concentrated carbohydrates - white bread, flour, cakes, pasta etc. made from refined flours. Most of the nutritional value has been removed and can have a negative effect on blood sugar levels.

Refined sugars - causes inflammatory reaction, produces a more acidic environment in the body which can increase the inflammation of endometriosis. Excessive amounts of acids are not at all good as they deplete oxygen, calcium and other minerals from your body. Refined sugar raises your blood sugar level quickly and this can cause insulin resistance. Insulin resistance has a major effect on your menstrual cycle. Sugar is also known to deplete your system of vitamins and minerals.

Caffeine - found in tea, coffee, soft drinks -increases abdominal cramps and caffeine increases estrogen levels. Coffee is also known to inhibit the absorption of iron. Caffeine also has a negative impact on our blood sugar level and is very toxic for our body. Furthermore, caffeine dehydrates the body and depletes vitamin B reserves.

Chocolate - (cheap commercial chocolate - as it contains sugar which is inflammatory, and unwanted additives) – *the good news* - organic dark chocolate is fine especially if it has high cacao content which has health benefits.

Dairy produce - including milk, cheese, butter, cream - cause inflammatory reaction as they increase the inflammatory prostaglandins. Dairy foods are also known to contain the second highest levels of dioxins. You may be OK with grass-fed butter or organic ghee, and an Elimination diet will let you know.

Eggs - advised to leave out eggs unless you can get organic as they may contain hormones. Soy is a common chicken feed and this can be transferred to eggs, which is another reason to only eat organic eggs.

Fried foods - can stimulate negative prostaglandins and can cause gut health issues as well as inflammation.

Saturated fats and oils – Foods that are high in fatty acids stimulate the negative inflammatory prostaglandins. Fatty acids are found in saturated fats, butter, margarine, lard.

Soy products and soy protein products - Soy is high in omega 6 which causes inflammation - tamari can be used in small amounts. Like wheat, soy contains phytic acid; however, the levels of phytic acid in soy are considerably higher than wheat. Phytic acid is known to irritate the digestive system and reduces mineral absorption, especially calcium. *More on soy further on.*

Convenience and processed foods - they contain a host of additives, cheap ingredients and have very little nutritional value. Processed foods can also increase negative prostaglandins.

Additives and preservatives - increases chemical load on the system especially your liver and your immune-system and have absolutely no nutritional value.

Alcohol - consumes vitamin B which is stored in the liver. Good liver function is vital as the liver will help to eliminate excess estrogen from the body. Alcohol also increases estrogen levels.

Some people require evidence and references to research regarding diet and endometriosis - you will find a PDF with links to research articles here:
https://www.endo-resolved.com/support-files/diet-endometriosis-link-research.pdf

Endometriosis & Estrogen In Your Diet

Endometriosis is fed by estrogen - this is well understood and documented. Women with endometriosis need to get their levels of estrogen to a natural balance along with progesterone, and other hormones.

Hormones are very powerful substances and it takes only microscopic amounts of any given hormone to activate a host of changes in the body.

It seems like an uphill battle to get the estrogen levels back into balance for women with endometriosis. Even men are being affected by the amount of estrogen in the environment with lower sperm counts and fertility problems. Children are beginning to enter puberty too early because of the estrogen in the environment. Wildlife is also being affected by estrogens that find their way into the environment.

Estrogens and estrogen mimics (xeno-estrogens) can be found in many sources including chemicals, toiletries, plastics, crop sprays, herbicides, canned foods, convenience foods and even found in several birth control pills.

Certain foods can mimic estrogens known as phyto-estrogens, but these are not as powerful or as damaging as other estrogen mimics. There are a few exceptions for those with endometriosis which are those foods that contain high levels of phyto-estrogens.

Highest sources of phyto-estrogenic foods:

All soy foods, flax seeds (very high levels), wheat bran, tofu, tempeh, miso paste

There are numerous other foods containing phyto-estrogens but many of them contain really low levels and will not cause issues if included in your diet.

What is interesting is that phyto-estrogens have been shown to have both estrogenic and anti-estrogenic effects. This means that, while some phyto-estrogens have estrogen-like effects and increase estrogen levels in your body, others block its effects and decrease estrogen levels. This means that having some phyto-estrgens in your diet can be beneficial, as long as you don't eat foods that contain high levels as this would be defeating the object of balancing these phyto-estrogens in your diet.

To protect yourself and balance your hormones:

- Avoid all foods that have been polluted and contain compounds and chemicals (xeno-estrogens) that act like estrogens in your body. These compounds are stored in body fat so will not be excreted out of your system.

- Avoid toiletries and cosmetics containing chemicals (xeno-estrogens) as they mimic estrogen. You also need to avoid toxic household cleaning products as these also contain harmful chemicals that can mimic estrogens.
- Include in your diet <u>some</u> foods that contain phyto-estrogens - but this must be done in a balanced way. The aim here is to take in phyto-estrogens so that they block the hormone pathways and stop your body absorbing negative estrogens.
- If you eat too many foods containing phyto-estrogens then you are defeating the object - you will end up with too much estrogen in your system. It is all about balance. Phyto-estrogens pose less of a threat to the body as they are much weaker and are not stored in the body.

Removing Estrogens With Diet

What if you have excess estrogens and have estrogen dominance?

Cruciferous vegetables are often suggested to help remove excess estrogens, which is a simple way to help balance your hormones. Cruciferous vegetables are rich in glucosinolates, which activate phase 2 detoxification in the liver, helping to filter estrogen metabolites from your body.

Cruciferous veggies that can remove estrogen including:

Broccoli, bok choy, brussels sprouts, kale, cabbage, cauliflower, and other leafy greens

Unfortunately, those with endometriosis may have a bad reaction to some of these veggies with bloating, gas and abdominal pain. The worse culprits tend to be cabbage and brussels sprouts. This is caused by the high levels of cellulose contained in these veggies which makes them harder to digest.

Cellulose is an insoluble fibre which will make it harder to breakdown and digest. The human body does not produce enzymes that are necessary to digest cellulose. When you consume cellulose, it passes through your stomach and small intestine undigested, and is eventually broken down by bacteria in the large intestine. They produce gases as a by-product of cellulose digestion, which is why high-fibre foods can sometimes cause bloating.

It is obviously going to be a good idea to be mindful of your reaction to these veggies. Don't go gung-ho and eat lots of veggies with the aim of removing estrogen from your body. You may end up trying to solve one problem only to end up with another. You need to keep track of your reaction and you can then avoid the ones that don't agree with you and cause gut distress. There are other ways to help remove excess estrogens with specific nutrients (which we cover later) as well as reducing your exposure to external estrogens from the environment (xeno-estrogens).

Eat This ...Not That...The Red Meat Debate

'Don't eat red meat' ... 'meat is not the problem' .... 'grass fed meat is OK'.
Constant conflicting information - let's have a look at some of the facts.

There are conflicting points of view as to whether red meat should be omitted from the diet to help with endometriosis. There are always two sides to a story and some say that eating grass-fed red meat is OK with endometriosis, but this is very individual.

Numerous research articles have found when women eat more red meat and processed meat, they tend to have a higher incidence of endometriosis. Additionally, there is powerful evidence and feedback from those with endometriosis, who say they feel so much better when they stop eating red meat.

There are several favourable arguments to stopping red meat when dealing with endometriosis and inflammation which include:

- Red meat can increase negative prostaglandins which are responsible for muscle cramping, uterine cramping, pain signals and inflammation.
- Red meat can increase levels of estrogen, and is often injected with hormones
- Additionally, meat contains natural estrogens, and can increase your own estrogen levels.
- There is little evidence to show that grass-fed meat is better for your estrogen levels. Cattle that are raised and fed as being grass-fed can still be given hay, haylage, silage and crop residue (which is open to speculation), so grass-fed cattle may not be as squeaky clean as promoted.
- Grass-fed beef is no longer regulated by governments in most countries and fake grass-fed meat is now entering the market.
- On top of that, most of the grass-fed beef sold at Walmart (USA) and other major chains is imported from Australia, Uruguay or other countries, but may still be labelled product of the USA. This begs the question, how is meat from another country to be regulated? 75% to 80% of grass-fed beef sold in the U.S. comes from abroad, according to reports.
- Due to the increased cost of raising cattle as grass-fed, the price of the meat can be as much as 70% higher, which encourages the market to be flooded with fake grass-fed meat.
- Red meat can be harder to digest which can cause problems for your digestive system and can cause bloating and gut pain. If you are feeling sluggish and tired after eating meat, it means you are not digesting it properly and you become drained of energy as your body is working hard to digest it.

Commercial meat issues

If you do not eat organic raised meat then eating commercially raised meat can be quite unhealthy, and I will not go into detail of the feed these poor cattle are given – it would turn your stomach.

- Current commercial farming and manufacturing practices in non-organic red meat can be full of hormones including estrogen, antibiotics and unwanted chemicals.
- Processed red meats are particularly harmful and commonly contain sodium, nitrates, phosphates and other food additives.
- Factory-farmed meats are high in certain endocrine disruptors and persistent organic pollutants (POPs).

Arachidonic Acid

Red meat contains arachidonic acid which is an omega 6 fatty acid and plays an important role in the inflammatory response. We do need these fatty acids as they play a vital role in ensuring our body responds properly to any physical damage or pathogen. However, having omega 6 fatty acid levels that are too high can upset the delicate balance of chemical pathways relating to pain and inflammation. It is worth noting that arachidonic acid is extremely high in grain fed meats, which is one good reason to ensure you only eat grass fed red meat.

Research

In the book '*The Endometriosis Health and Diet Program*', Dr Cook and Danielle Cook state that all meat and dairy contain dioxins due to the build-up in the environment, and they suggest keeping meat consumption to a limited amount. Additionally, there is one study (*Selected Food Intake and Risk of Endometriosis - F Parazzin., 2004*) that found women who ate a diet high in red meat and ham had a significant increase of endometriosis.

Endometriosis, iron and red meat

It is understandable that women with endometriosis feel the need to eat red meat due to suffering anaemia caused by heavy periods. However, there are other food sources of iron including: cashew nuts, kidney beans, pumpkin seeds, sesame seeds, hemp seeds, oats, quinoa, spinach, dark chocolate, blackstrap molasses, lentils, chickpeas, and kale.

The take-away to this advice – if you can guarantee that the meat you purchase is organic grass-fed meat AND it causes you no problems with symptoms of pain or having a flare, then you are obviously OK to eat red meat.

'One wo-man's meat is another wo-man's poison'

So, What Can You Eat?

We covered earlier the foods you are advised to leave out of your diet, but what can you actually eat? Your diet needs to be well balanced to provide a varied and nutritious diet, and eating regular meals throughout the day to help keep your blood sugars balanced.

Here are suggestions to include in your diet

White meat - chicken and turkey – aim to eat organic – obviously plenty of dishes can be made with white meats like curries, casseroles, grilled chicken etc.

Oily fish - rich in omega 3 oils which can help to reduce inflammation and pain. Best options are salmon, mackerel, sardines, herring and trout.

Gluten free foods - instead of wheat based - many supermarkets are now stocking lots of gluten free breads, savoury biscuits, gluten free breakfast cereals etc.

Lots of veg based meals - add in pulses to veg based meals and you will obtain plenty of nutrition and as well as protein. This will help support a healthy gut microbiome as well as reduce estrogen in your system.

Fruit - great for making smoothies and you can add in extra nutrients with protein powders and other super-foods. Try not to overdo it on your fruit consumption due to fruit sugars but one or two portions a day is OK as part of a balanced diet.

For carbs - your options include rice, rice noodles, gluten free oats, quinoa as well as beans and pulses. These are complex carbs which will help to sustain your blood sugar levels.

For pasta dish options - using gluten free pasta, or you can use spiralized veggies like zucchini instead of pasta.

Baked items - try to limit these but you can have breads, cakes, cookies etc, using gluten free flour. Try to reserve these items for the occasional treat.

Desserts – you will find many recipes online that are sugar, gluten and dairy free.

Nuts, dried fruits and seeds - nuts are good for snacking, seeds are full of nutrients and can be sprinkled on many dishes.

Alternative milks - almond milk, cashew milk, oat milk, rice milk and coconut milk

Herb teas - peppermint tea is good for nausea; chamomile is ideal as an evening tea to help calm you down and aid with sleep.

You will find plenty of anti-inflammatory recipes online and Pinterest is a good resource. Also, there are numerous anti-inflammatory cookbooks available which will provide recipes for most of your diet needs.

At times we tend to focus more on all the things we CAN'T eat rather than all the things we CAN eat. If you're saying to yourself 'no, I can't eat this, and I can't eat that', it's going to make you feel stuck and not enjoy being healthy. This mindset is what makes you want to eat more of what is bad for you.

Don't Feel Like Cooking?

There will be times when you don't feel like cooking. You are too tired, too sick, feeling weak and just don't want to be stood in the kitchen cooking food. All you really want to do is curl up on the couch under a blanket with a hot water bottle and a cup of tea.

But you need to eat ... period! You need to keep your blood sugars stable, and your body needs the nutrients for it to work and to heal. I put the question to women with endometriosis on a few message boards asking what they eat when they don't feel like cooking and had some helpful responses.

These were some of the suggestions:

- Soups – soups came out as top of the list from the feedback. There are so many recipes for veggie soups and you will find endless recipe ideas online. The best approach is to batch cook and freeze a few portions for those days you don't feel like cooking.
- Batch cooking and freezing meals – like casseroles, mild curries, pasta sauces etc.
- Ready-prepped veggie burgers, patties that have been frozen served with salad
- Salad with some protein like a piece of grilled fish or left-over cooked chicken
- Add sprouted seeds and grains to your meals for extra nutrition
- Baked sweet potato with salad
- Natural yogurt with chopped fruit, nuts or seeds
- Oatmeal topped with fruit
- Oatcakes and nut butter
- GF toast with dips, hummus etc.
- Chia pudding with fruit
- Smoothies – you can add all sorts of nutrients like hemp seeds, protein power
- Hummus or dips with crackers

Endo Friendly Snack Ideas

When dealing with endometriosis it seems common to have a regular case of the munchies. We need to keep our blood sugars balanced and a healthy snack can stop those sudden blood sugar drops. I personally think that the need for regular snacks is caused by the body working so hard to 'manage' the disease and the immune system is dealing with a heavy work load.

Keeping your blood sugars stable with health snacks will take the stress off your system and help sustain your energy.

Here are a few healthy snack ideas to keep you going:

- Dried fruit and nut mix
- Hummus or dips with gluten free crackers
- Fruit and nut protein bars
- Protein/power balls
- Rice crackers with dips
- Fruit - plain and simple
- Yoghurt mixed with chopped fruit, nuts and seeds
- Apple slices with peanut butter or almond butter
- Home-made gluten free, sugar free muffins
- Sweet potato crackers
- Dark chocolate - the higher the cacao content the better for nutrition
- Gluten free oatcakes with dips/peanut butter
- Smoothies with added chia seeds for nutrition, energy and to fill you up
- Diced/sliced avocado with tahini dressing

Soy & Endometriosis

I want to quickly cover the topic of soy in your diet – it's one of my pet topics regarding endometriosis and diet! Sometimes when people change their diet and stop eating meat, they often start to eat soy-based alternative products.

Soy is found in dozens of items: granola, vegetarian chilli, a vast sundry of imitation animal foods, pasta, most protein powders and 'power' bars, soy milk, soy yoghurts, soy-based cheeses, to name just a few.

I always advise women to stop eating soy and the feedback I receive from women is always positive with an improvement in their symptoms.

Why is it advised to not eat soy?

It sometimes seems to be unclear for some why soy should be omitted from the diet when you have endometriosis. In principle soy products will upset your natural hormone balance because soy contains **high** levels of phyto-estrogens which will mimic your own estrogen hormones.

Having *some* phyto-estrogens in our diet can be beneficial, as we have covered, as they are thought to block our estrogen receptors and help to reduce excess estrogens from circulating in our system. But having too many phyto-estrogens can tip the balance.

However, the problem with soy goes beyond the issue of phyto-estrogens. Soy can cause many negative health problems which seems to be worse for those with endometriosis.

Some of these problems include:

- Causing hormone imbalances
- Can cause serious disruption in thyroid hormone levels
- High levels of omega 6 which can cause inflammation
- High levels of phytic acid in soy reduce assimilation of calcium, magnesium, copper, iron and zinc
- Levels of soy phyto-estrogens disrupt endocrine function
- Soy foods contain high levels of aluminium which is toxic to the nervous system and the kidneys, and can also cause problems with the thyroid
- Soy foods increase the body's requirement for vitamin D
- The various negative effects of soy weaken the immune system.
- Ninety one percent of the soy grown in the United States is genetically engineered and **is regularly sprayed with pesticides** - all of which are detrimental to health
- Soy cultivation is also bad for the environment - in the space of about half an hour, an area of Brazil's Amazon rainforest larger than 200 football fields will have been destroyed, much of it for soybean cultivation, most of which is fed to livestock.

Phytic Acid and Soy

Phytic acid has been highlighted by Dian Mills in her book '*Endometriosis - Healing through Diet and Nutrition*', as being a particularly problematic compound that is found in wheat. She speculates that it is the phytic acid in wheat which aggravates the symptoms of endometriosis. Phytic acid is found at higher levels in soy than it is in wheat, which as mentioned is detrimental for your health and will reduce absorption of vital nutrients.

Please do not eat soy as it has many harmful effects on your health

Plant Sources Of Protein

If you decide to go totally plant based with your diet, then you obviously need to be eating alternative sources of proteins.

You need to ensure you have protein in your diet as protein contains amino acids that aid in healing. Also, protein is needed to support healthy neurotransmitter production as well as build healthy muscles.

Examples of vegetarian foods with high sources of protein:

Protein in legumes/grains: Legumes- also called dried beans are edible seeds that grow in pods. Beans contain a more complete set of amino acids than other plant-based food and they are high in iron, B vitamins and fibre.

Use legumes as main dish items rather than side dishes. A good way to introduce beans to the diet is to replace the meat component in your favourite dishes, like casseroles, chilli, curries, and adding beans to salad dishes. Examples are chickpeas or garbanzo beans, split peas, haricot, lentils (red, green or brown), kidney beans, lima beans etc.

Protein in grains: Whole grains are an excellent source of nutrition, as they contain essential enzymes, iron, dietary fibre, vitamin E, and the B-complex vitamins. Because the body absorbs grain slowly, they provide sustained and high-quality energy. Grains can be added to casseroles or used in a side dish. Examples are: brown rice, buckwheat, millet, oatmeal, quinoa, wild rice

Vegetable protein: Nutritionally, greens are very high in protein, calcium, magnesium, iron, potassium, phosphorous, zinc, and vitamins A, C, E and K. They are crammed with fibre, folic acid, chlorophyll and many other micro-nutrients. Simply stir-fry or steam some broccoli, kale, bok choy, or cabbage to get a good fix on nutrients as well as proteins.

Protein in nuts and seeds: Nuts are very healthy and nutritious. In addition to being excellent sources of protein, nuts and seeds have other nutrients such as vitamins, minerals, fibre, and other micro-nutrients that may prevent cancer and heart disease. Additionally, nuts are high in essential amino acids and healthy fats and essential fatty acids (omega 3). Nuts and seeds can be added to salads as well as eaten as a snack. The most common nuts and seeds include almonds, cashews, pumpkin seeds, sesame seeds, sunflower seeds, walnuts.

Alternative Ingredients For Your Diet

You will be needing to replace certain ingredients in your diet, especially for those foods you have found are your particular triggers.

The main food groups you will be looking for alternative ingredients will be **dairy, wheat and sugar.**

Milk alternatives

The best milk alternatives include:

- Almond milk
- Rice milk
- Coconut milk
- Cashew milk
- Oat milk

Most of these are easy to find in your health food store and many supermarkets are starting to supply different dairy alternatives. Just make sure not to use soy milk. You also need to be careful not to purchase coconut milk containing carrageenan as it can trigger an inflammatory response in the body.

Sugar alternatives

This can be a hard one for most to give up but there are other options to add sweetness to your cooking. Stevia is a good all-round sweetener and readily available to purchase. Other sweeteners may be suggested in specific recipes for desserts and for baked items, and sometimes the choice of sweetener is made to help add extra moisture to a recipe.

Alternative sweeteners include:

- Amsake
- Brown rice syrup
- Date sugar
- Honey
- Maple syrup
- Stevia

Wheat alternatives

Many different gluten free flours can be used instead of wheat for making breads, pastries, muffins and so on. You may need to experiment to find the flour blend and recipes that suit you and you will find many recipes online.

Flours that are gluten free:

- Amaranth flour – often used in baking
- Buckwheat flour – slightly nutty taste
- Corn-flour – used for thickening sauces
- Chickpea flour – slightly nutty taste
- Potato flour – this is a very heavy flour
- Quinoa flour – provides a plant source of protein
- White rice flour – ideal for recipes that require a light texture

Many health shops will supply alternative ingredients and even supermarkets are now selling healthy options for many ingredients. Most supermarkets these days also provide a line in gluten free options including ready meals and frozen meals. Obtaining healthy ingredient options is getting easier and if your local supermarket does not have what you are looking for then there are always plenty of options online.

Recipes

Initially, this book was going to include a collection of anti-inflammatory recipes BUT the book was becoming longer and longer. I really wanted this book to focus on natural treatments and self-help remedies and not get diverted into becoming another recipe book. So …. I decided a way round this was to offer you a separate e-book of recipes you can download.

The recipes are all anti-inflammatory using safe alternative ingredients and include energy bite/snack recipes, smoothies, salads, healing soups, collection of mains recipes, desserts, dip recipes and finally an endo-friendly chocolate recipe- yay!

You will find your download for the e-book here:

https://www.endo-resolved.com/support-files/healing-book-complimentary-recipes.pdf

'If you feel like giving up because
you are not seeing results, remember this;
The last thing to grow on a fruit tree is the fruit' - Anon

Additional

Nutrition

Tips

'We know that food is a medicine, perhaps the most powerful drug on the planet with the power to cause or cure most disease.'

Dr Mark Hyman

Use The Right Oils In Your Diet

The types of oils you use in your diet with endometriosis are important

Certain oils can affect your symptoms as they react in your body and can cause inflammation as well increase your pain – remember the topic of prostaglandins and pain.

Processed vegetable oils are really bad for you. During the extraction process of many oils, they undergo a heat and/or chemical process to remove the oil from the seed and to clarify and deodorise it. This process completely changes the molecular structure and in turn the body will treat it as a chemical.

It then has to be eliminated from the body by the liver by manufacturing specific enzymes. If your body's metabolism is compromised in any way, like disease, this will cause further ill health issues.

The only vegetable oils to eat are those which have been produced by being cold-pressed during the processing. The best oils for you to be using are natural, unrefined cold-pressed oils. They need to belong to the group of oils that contain essential fatty acids of omega 3 which are anti-inflammatory.

These can be found in: olive oil, walnut oil, avocado oil

Cooking with oils

Just as you need to be careful which oils you use with endometriosis, (or any inflammatory disease) you need to know which oils to use when cooking, as certain oils become degraded during cooking, and particular oils are best when used cold, as in salad dressings.

For high temperatures

When it comes to cooking at high temperatures coconut oils is a clear winner. With more than 90 percent of its fatty acids being saturated fats, this makes coconut oil super heat resistant. Many are concerned when they hear that coconut oil is high in saturated fats which increases cholesterol.

However, coconut oil contains both lauric acid which raises LDL (or bad cholesterol), but it also increases HDL (good cholesterol) dramatically. The lauric acid in coconut oil can help reduce Candida infection in the gut, it is reported to be anti-inflammatory, and has antibacterial, antifungal and antiviral properties.

Although this oil is semi-solid at average room temperatures, it turns liquid very quickly when warmed up. Coconut oil can be stored for years in a sealed container and never go rancid. To get the most health benefits possible, always choose virgin coconut oil.

Another good oil to use for cooking at high temperatures is avocado oil, and as it does not have much taste many prefer this oil for cooking.

Oils to use at medium-low heat

First cold pressed unrefined olive oil, avocado oil and almond oil are good choices. Store the oil in glass airtight bottles in a cool, dark place. Use within two months of opening.

Oils to use cold only

First cold pressed, unrefined hemp oil, walnut oil and sesame seed oil are all good options. Walnut oil is a good source of important nutrients, including B vitamins, vitamin E, selenium, iron, and calcium and walnut oil may even help stabilize hormone levels. Store in small dark glass airtight bottles in the back of the refrigerator. Use within one month of opening. These oils are ideal for making salad dressings.

Oils to avoid

Unfortunately, most of the oils on the market today are industrial seed, GMO, highly processed vegetable oils. These oils are very bad for your health as they are loaded with omega-6 fatty acids, which can cause inflammation – not to mention the toxic affects they have on your liver as well as containing chemical residue from processing the oils. One of the most common chemicals used in oil extraction is hexane, which is a by-product from gasoline production, which is a serious neurotoxin.

The oils you need to avoid include safflower oil, soybean oil, rice bran oil, corn oil, cottonseed oil, sunflower oil, canola oil and rapeseed oil. Be careful where you obtain your advice as I have seen websites recommending these oils as being safe for cooking – but they are not.

Dietary Nutrients & Supplements

The use of dietary supplements must go hand in hand with a healthy anti-inflammatory diet. It is not enough to take supplements and continue with poor dietary habits. I have observed that some women have tried different supplements and not changed their diet and have wondered why they are not seeing any improvements.

Often diet alone cannot provide all the nutrients you require for optimal health. This can be caused by poor soil quality which means vital nutrients are now missing in the food that is grown today. Modern food production has become far removed from the foods our ancestors used to eat.

Topping up your needs with certain supplements will ensure your body obtains the nutrients it needs. The following list of nutritional supplements will help to support various bodily processes and can also help with certain symptoms of endometriosis.

B vitamins - these are important for the breakdown of proteins, carbohydrates and fats in the body. Vitamin B6 is particularly helpful as this vitamin can **help to regulate estrogen levels**. As well as supplementing, B vitamins can be found in bee pollen which is easily added to your diet in smoothies or your morning oats**.**

B12 - Vitamin B12 is needed for producing and maintaining new cells, including nerve cells and red blood cells. Those who stop eating meat or who have any intestinal disorders that interfere with absorption may need to take a vitamin B12 supplement. Methyl-cobalamin is a natural, active form of vitamin B12 and one that is more easily absorbed. It is advised to use sublingual forms as this bypass the gut and is absorbed directly into the blood-stream. Foods rich in vitamin B12 include sardines, tuna, herring, mackerel and trout.

Vitamin C - is well known for helping to boost the immune system and help provide resistance to disease. Vitamin C is also able **to help inhibit negative prostaglandins** responsible for causing pain and inflammation. A great source of vitamin C can be found in camu-camu powder, citrus fruits, broccoli, kale and other green veggies.

Calcium - levels of calcium in menstruating women decrease 10 to 14 days before the onset of menstruation. Deficiency may lead to muscle cramps, headache or pelvic pain. When stopping dairy in your diet you need to look at alternative sources of calcium which can be found in sesame seeds, kale, almonds, broccoli and sweet potatoes.

Carnitine - Carnitine is an amino acid that improves energy levels by transporting fatty acids into the mitochondria where they can be burned up and used as fuel. Carnitine boosts energy, improves brain and cognitive function and can regulate blood sugar.

Carnitine is found mainly in dairy and red meats, and I always advise those I work with to supplement with carnitine when they have removed these foods. Carnitine is easily found in supplement form as a powder and can be mixed into smoothies/juices/soups.

Vitamin D - Vitamin D is an interesting one as it actually a hormone belonging to the steroid family. Women with endometriosis can be low in Vitamin D, and one study has shown that woman are actually already low in this vital vitamin/hormone. If you are not getting sufficient sunlight there is a good chance your vitamin D can be low and supplementing daily will help. Vitamin D needs to be taken at the same time as a high fat meal and is better taken earlier in the day as some find vitamin D can be stimulating

Vitamin E - plays an important role by increasing oxygen carrying capacities and also strengthens the immune system. Vitamin E is able to help inhibit the negative prostaglandins and is also helpful for reducing estrogen levels in the body. A study published in Pubmed suggested that natural antioxidants such as vitamin E and C at low doses, are an effective alternative therapy to relieve chronic pelvic pain in women with endometriosis.

Iron - as we have noted, women with endometriosis tend to have very heavy periods which can lead to an iron deficiency. This can lead to anaemia which is characterized by extreme fatigue and weakness. As well as supplementing with grass-fed beef liver, you can also increase your iron levels with Blackstrap Molasses.

Magnesium - is a mineral we can easily become depleted in, often due to stress. Magnesium can ease cramping with menstruation and is a great muscle relaxant. It also assists with maintaining water levels in the gut and can help with the problem of constipation. If you want to increase your magnesium with diet, the foods high in magnesium include cacao, nuts and leafy greens.

Omega 3 oils - this is one key supplement you are advised to include in your diet as omega 3 helps to reduce pain, reduce inflammation as well as reduce the bad prostaglandins that cause pain. Eating a couple of portions of oily fish a week will help as well as taking a daily supplement.

Selenium - Selenium is a mineral that can be depleted due to poor soil which is now low in selenium levels. When selenium is taken together with vitamin E it has been reported to decrease inflammation associated with endometriosis, as well as being an immune system booster. Selenium can also support thyroid function, but be careful not to overdo it when supplementing Selenium as too much can be toxic.

A Special Note About Iron

As we have already noted, women with endometriosis often suffer from anaemia due to heavy blood loss. Let's have a closer look at the effects of low iron and anaemia as you may be thinking your fatigue is purely down to your endometriosis. Anaemia is a deficiency of iron in the body. Iron helps your body replenish red blood cells and a vital role is to transport oxygen to your tissues throughout your body.

Reasons why iron is important

- Iron carries oxygen from your tissues to your lungs, so if your iron is low it will show up as breathlessness and your heart-rate has to go up in response to less oxygen.
- Iron also directly helps with energy production by driving the electron transport chain, or ETC -- a series of chemical reactions that help you get energy from carbohydrates, proteins and fats.
- Iron improves your immune system, which means if your iron is low, you are more susceptible to infections and illness.

- Iron helps raise dopamine and serotonin in your brain, and low iron can leave you feeling depressed.
- Iron assists with promoting cortisol secretion and if your iron is low, then cortisol secretion is decreased as well as lowering glucose in your cells.
- Iron promotes good conversion of thyroid hormones T4 to T3 (the active hormone) which is important for those with a thyroid problem.
- If iron is low your T4 will build too high which will leave you feeling rather toxic.
- Iron balances your autonomic nervous system, so with low iron you can end up in a frequent state of fight-or-flight with accompanying adrenaline surges and nervousness due to heightened sympathetic activity.
- Low Iron affects brain cell health, so if your iron is low, you can have brain cell death contributing to dementia and possibly Alzheimer's.

Symptoms of iron deficiency include:

- Weakness
- Pale Skin
- Cold hands and feet
- Bruising easily
- Headaches
- Dizziness, or an overall feeling of light-headedness
- Poor appetite
- Breathlessness

Some with endometriosis have tried iron supplements due to confirmed very low iron (with blood tests) and have found them ineffective. Often this can be remedied by taking vitamin C at the same time as iron, as vitamin C aids in absorption of iron.

A gentle and safe way to increase your iron intake is with grass-fed beef liver capsules or Blackstrap Molasses, and you should be able to restore your iron balance within 3 to 4 weeks if your iron depletion is not too serious.

Those who have had successfully reduced their symptoms by stopping red meat may worry about becoming low in iron, but there are many other sources or iron you can obtain through diet including lentils, beans, leafy vegetables, pumpkin, sesame and hemp seeds, oats, nuts and nut butters especially almonds and cashew nuts.

The dried herb of thyme also has good levels of iron and thyme has additional benefits for mood and brain health. Thyme is a great source of lithium and tryptophan and both can help as mood stabilizers and aid sleep. Thyme makes a great tea, especially when added to peppermint.

If you feel any of the above symptoms that describe iron deficiency, please consult with your doctor before taking any iron supplements. A full iron-panel blood test is required to assess your total iron status, which includes:

TIBC - Total iron-binding capacity (TIBC), Transferrin saturation, Ferritin and UBIC (Unsaturated iron binding capacity).

Once you have tested your iron levels you will then know how to proceed and your doctor may suggest supplementing if your iron levels are very low.

Foods To Support Your System

As a major issue with endometriosis is related to inflammation, then cutting out inflammatory foods as we have covered, is a prime way to help with this problem. To aid the healing process and help reduce inflammation further you can add in foods that are known to be anti-inflammatory.

Here is a run-down of different foods that have anti-inflammatory properties including fats, spices/herbs, veggies, grains/pulses and fruits. I have also included in this list plant sources of natural pain-killers, plant sources of omega 3, as well as foods to support your immune-system – just to give you an extra nutritional boost.

Anti-inflammatory foods to include in your diet

Feel free to include any of these anti-inflammatory foods in your diet. The only exception to this list is for those who have done an elimination diet and found any of these foods cause a bad reaction, then you obviously need to remove them from your diet. One of the main problem foods can be vegetables with a high cellulose content, especially when eaten raw, but when cooked, these foods can often be OK and not cause problems – just keep a track of what you eat and you will learn what you can and cannot eat.

Anti-inflammatory Fats - Almonds, Avocados, Brazil nuts, Cashews, Chia seeds, Hazelnuts, Hemp seeds, Olives, Peanuts, Pecans, Pistachios, Sesame seeds, Sunflower seeds

Anti-inflammatory Herbs/Spices - Basil, Cayenne pepper, Cilantro/coriander, Cinnamon, Cloves, Cumin, Curry, Dill, Ginger, Garlic, Mint, Oregano, Parsley, Rosemary, Sage, Thyme, Turmeric

Anti-inflammatory Grains - Amaranth, Brown Rice, Buckwheat, Bulgar, Millet, Oats, Quinoa, Wild Rice

Anti-inflammatory Beans & Pulses - Adzuki Beans, Black Beans, Cannellini Beans, Garbanzo/chickpea Beans, Green Beans, Lentils, Butter Beans, Navy Beans

Anti-inflammatory Starchy Vegetables - Squash, Potatoes, Parsnips, Pumpkin, Yams

Anti-inflammatory Vegetables - Broccoli, Cabbage, Carrots, Cauliflower, Celery, Cucumber, Eggplant/Aubergine, Garlic, Lettuce, Kale, Leeks, Onion, Peppers - all types, Shallots, Spinach, Tomato, Watercress, Zucchini/courgette

* As well as being anti-inflammatory, the high fibre in veggies will help to remove excess estrogen from your system

Anti-inflammatory Fruit - Apple, Banana, Blackberries, Blueberries, Cherries, Dates, Grapes, Melon, Lemon, Mango, Orange, Papaya, Pineapple, Plum, Strawberries, Watermelon

Plant based natural painkillers

Ginger, turmeric, garlic, pineapple, peppermint, horseradish, chilli, carrots, cayenne pepper, grapes, oats, cherries.

These are all good natural pain killers to include in your diet. Oats can be eaten daily for breakfast, peppermint makes a really tasty tea that is really effective for reducing nausea, and turmeric is used by many with great effect to reduce pain and inflammation.

Note * There are some studies that say turmeric can affect the absorption of iron, so please be mindful as it may affect your iron levels. If taking turmeric, it is best to avoid taking it with meals rich in iron if you are aiming to keep your iron levels up.

Plant sources of omega 3

Chia seeds, sunflower seeds, hemp hearts/hemp oil, avocado, avocado oil, leafy greens, winter squash, walnuts, walnut oil, walnut butter, wild rice, kidney beans, seaweed, nori, algae oil (found in supplements), flax seeds (but these are high in estrogen so need to be limited). And of course, oily fish is high in omega 3's.

Foods Beneficial For The Immune System

A key component of managing endometriosis is about supporting your immune system and certain foods are very helpful for this function. Most of these foods are easy to add into your diet on a daily basis.

- Coconut Oil - add a spoonful to your morning oats
- Green tea - have one or two cups a day (in between meals)

- Garlic (raw or lightly cooked) - add to your favourite savoury dishes
- Pineapple (contains bromelain which is anti-inflammatory) - add to a morning smoothie
- Carrots (contain beta-carotene) - try diced roasted carrots mixed with other root veggies. Carrots also contain a natural pain-killing compound
- Live yoghurt (to obtain healthy bacteria) - add to your morning smoothie blend
- Seeds: sesame, pumpkin, chia, hemp - add to smoothies, stir into soup, sprinkle on the top of dishes
- Sprouted seed - increases nutritional value by 2000%
- Red/purple berries- eat any way you like and add some live yoghurt
- Ginger - use fresh chopped ginger and steep in hot water for 10 minutes, add honey and drink
- Elderberry - drink the juice just as it comes
- Kidney Beans, peas, lentils - can be added to many savoury dishes

Control Stable Blood Sugar Levels

Maintaining stable blood sugar levels is
vital to help control hormones in your body

Controlling your blood sugars means eating in a way that stops the blood sugar roller coaster, where your blood sugar and insulin spikes and crashes continuously, which can lead to many hormone imbalances.

- When you eat the wrong foods, like sugary foods, you end up with an insulin spike, and when you have too much insulin it can cause other hormones to go out of whack. This can then lead to an increase in cortisol.
- Cortisol can compete with progesterone, and cortisol usually takes precedence over progesterone. This then leads to a reduction of progesterone and can cause estrogen dominance.
- Additionally, there are insulin receptors on the ovaries and excess insulin causes the ovaries to produce more male hormones as opposed to the necessary female hormones, which can lead to issues like PCOS.

As you can see – everything in the body has a knock-on effect and you have to be very mindful of what you put in your body as it affects so many systems, including your hormones.

Blood sugars and brain health

Blood sugars not only affect your energy level, weight, inflammation levels, and thyroid function, they also affect how your brain functions.

Glucose is the brain's fuel source, making stable blood sugar vital to healthy, balanced brain chemistry and the prevention of neurodegeneration. When blood sugar is unstable – either too high or too low – not enough glucose gets to the brain and the brain will degenerate and not function well.

Here are a few tips to help stabilise blood sugar levels:

- Include fat/protein with every meal: nuts, seeds, fish, healthy oils like coconut oil
- Eat every three to four hours with small healthy snacks between meals if needed
- Reduce fruit juice intake or combine fruit juice with vegetable juice in smoothies
- Eat breakfast within one hour of waking
- Aim to include protein with breakfast
- Avoid foods with high glycaemic index
- Always combine carbohydrates with fat or protein
- Reduce simple carbs and ensure you focus on complex carbs
- Try teaspoon of natural peanut butter/nut butter before bed to sustain blood sugar levels over night

Breakfast to stabilize blood sugars

Eating breakfast is the most important meal of the day to stabilize blood sugar levels, and most importantly, eating good quality protein and fat. You have been fasting for hours while asleep and your adrenal glands are now working overtime to make up for low blood sugars. Now is the time to feed your adrenals, feed your body with nutrients and sustain blood sugar levels.

You may wake up with no appetite or suffer nausea and this is a side effect of your adrenal hormones, and using caffeine will only make matters worse, so try to eat some protein, even if is only a small amount. After a few days, this will start to stabilize your blood sugars.

Good & Bad Carbs & Blood Sugars

Controlling your blood sugars will depend on the type of carbs you eat

Carbs are carbohydrates which are sugars and starches which are responsible for providing a major part of the energy that our body needs. When we eat carbohydrates, our body converts them into glycogen which provides the energy we need to function.

Good carbs:

- Good carbs are more complex and provide slow and steady energy
- Good carbohydrates are rich in minerals, nutrients and vitamins.
- Keeps you feeling fuller for longer
- Provide natural sugars so does not spike blood sugars
- Higher fibre content

Sources: whole grains, vegetables, legumes

Bad carbs

- Digested very quickly so can leave you feeling hungry sooner
- Can cause sugar cravings
- Spikes blood sugar levels
- Can convert to fat easily
- Low fibre content
- Contain higher levels of saturated fats

Sources: processed foods, refined baked goods and bread, refined grains

The problem with bad carbs is that most of us love the taste of foods that are made of bad carbs. You just have to think of pizza, baked goods, desserts, cakes … the list goes on. The solution is to find recipes using alternative healthy ingredients, which are compiled to give you tasty options so that you don't feel like you are missing out on the foods you use to enjoy.

You will find many recipes online that are gluten, dairy and sugar free that provide many tasty alternatives. As well as the complimentary recipe e-book, you will find some more recipes at the website at endo-resolved and Pinterest is also a good place for recipes.

Going Gluten Free

Many with endometriosis respond well to going gluten free to help reduce their symptoms, especially bloating and inflammation

What exactly is gluten

Gluten is found in many sources and not only in food, but the most common source of gluten is found in wheat and many with endometriosis respond well to going gluten free.

Gluten is the general name for one of the proteins found in wheat, rye, and barley. It is the substance in flour that forms the structure of dough, and is the 'glue' that holds the product together, and is also the leavening ingredient.

Endometriosis is an inflammatory disease and gluten can make inflammation worse by the way it acts on the gut. Part of the aim of treating endometriosis naturally is to help reduce inflammation, so avoiding anything that contains gluten will help.

In one endometriosis study 75% of participants reported a significant improvement in their symptoms after going gluten free for 12 months

The wheat crop has been extensively genetically modified over time. This genetic modification has in turn altered the structure of gluten, which has led it to becoming hybridized to create new protein structures that the human body has a hard time breaking down. This can then trigger inflammation.

Where is gluten found?

Gluten is mainly found in grains including wheat, rye, barley, and all their derivatives. These grains are used in such items as breads, cereals, pasta, pizza, cakes, pies, and cookies and as added ingredients to many processed food items.

Gluten can also be found in bulgar, couscous, durum wheat, rye, kamut, and spelt. You also need to watch out for wheat-bran, wheat-germ and wheat-starch.

Gluten can also be found in the following:

Ales, beer and lagers, brown rice syrup, pasta, sauces, soup base, stuffing, imitation bacon/seafood, marinades and thickeners, soy sauce, herbal supplements, vitamin and mineral supplements.

Be sure to read all labels carefully. If a product has questionable ingredients, avoid it. Remember wheat free, does not mean gluten free. Look for words 'wheat, barley, rye, malt' on labels to identify if there is any gluten present.

Tips for going gluten free

Going gluten free may not always seem straight forward especially when you read all the places that gluten can be found. Here are a few pointers to help you make the change.

Swop out your current gluten containing ingredients and change them for gluten free options but be sure not to buy alternatives that are laden with additives, preservatives and especially watch out for soy.

One of the hardest things to swop is changing to gluten free bread, as they are not always that tasty. However, you do not always have to use bread to make sandwiches. You can use gluten free pitta bread; tortilla wraps and rice crackers.

- Many food producers now make gluten free pastas and you can use rice noodles instead of wheat-based noodles
- Aim for simple meals which are obviously gluten free, like white meats, fish, vegetables, fruits, pulses, nuts.
- Check out the GF sections at your supermarket and local health store to see what they have to offer
- Always check your labels to ensure you are not getting any hidden gluten
- Swop your Soy sauce for Tamari or Coconut Aminos (an alternative to soy)
- Many supplement and vitamin manufacturers are aware of gluten and allergy issues so check you are buying from reliable sources
- If you are going to eat out at a restaurant give them a ring first to check they have gluten free options

Buying GF foods

As the demand for GF products increases, many grocery stores and supermarkets are now beginning to stock more products that are specifically gluten-free. Look in the Asian section for rice noodles and crackers. Check out the 'organic' or 'health food' section for GF pastas, flours, and baking products.

You need to be aware that many gluten free 'alternative' products like breads and ready meals are processed and are not particularly nutritious, especially the ones with corn and white rice flower. You also need to avoid those with sugar and unnatural additives. Try not to focus on gluten free products too much, it's better to change your way of eating. Go for pure, natural, wholefoods.

But you can make use of the healthy gluten free options so that you can increase your dietary choices.

Eating Organic

If at all possible, try to eat organic. This applies not only to fruit, vegetables and meat, but to other produce as well. You will find an increasing number of food stores and supermarkets who are beginning to supply a wide range of organic produce.

This can include organic rice, pulses, different flours, nuts, canned foods, frozen foods - in fact most foods can be purchased these days that are organic. Many people think of shopping for organic food only for fresh produce, but today there are many different healthy organic foods available.

OK, it may be more expensive to purchase organic foods, but you can make savings by not eating those expensive convenience foods. As the number of organic growers increases the cost of organic foods will continue to drop, and in summer you could always grow your own salads and veggies. If you have a south facing window you can grow salad greens on your windowsill.

If you are going to include meat in your diet, it is best that it comes from an organic farm, where the live-stock has been raised and fed organically.

Added to this, I advise you to try and purchase from local organic growers and check your local Farmers Markets. There have been some unscrupulous practises uncovered where growers/distributors are importing their produce, which has been found to be far from organic because of the use of sprays and chemicals.

It stands to reason that any foods which are going to be put into storage and then shipped around the world will have to be treated in some way to stop it rotting. It does not bare thinking about. Some of your food may have even been gassed - especially if it is going to be in storage for months while it is shipped. The bottom line - try and purchase from your local growers, and you will be supporting local business, reducing your food miles as well as helping your local economy.

Fibre In Your Diet

Fibre (yes, that's the way we spell it in my neck of the woods!) plays a very important role in maintaining a healthy digestive system. Having a good fibre balance in your diet will help to alleviate constipation and will also help to flush excess estrogens from the body.

The best source of dietary fibre is from whole foods, unrefined wholegrain cereals, nuts, seeds, berries and pulses. Fibrous vegetables like celery, carrot, potato and other root vegetables and legumes are also good sources of dietary fibre.

Let's clear up any 'grey areas' regarding fibre and constipation!

There are two types of fibre – soluble and non-soluble – and you need to eat a balance of the two. The non-soluble fibre is found in the rough part of foods – the husks of grain, the skins of certain fruits and vegetables. The soluble fibre is found in higher amounts in fruit and vegetables as well as in legumes.

The words soluble or non-soluble refer to whether a fibre is dissolved and broken down in your system. If you eat mainly non-soluble fibre you could end up being MORE constipated because this type of fibre will absorb water from your gut as it goes through the digestive system.

On the other hand, if you eat lots of soluble fibre then you could end up with 'the runs'. So please balance your fibre between the two types to stop any issues of constipation developing. So many doctors simply say .. 'Are you getting enough fibre', without explaining that you need to eat a balance of both types.

If you stuff yourself with brown rice you will just clog yourself up!

Superfoods To Support Your System

Superfoods are an easy way to get a nutritional boost into your diet and are preferable to taking lots of supplements to support your nutritional needs. Superfoods comprise a diverse collection of nutrient-rich natural foods such as berries, seeds, grains, algae, vegetables and fruits, with most of them having much higher nutritional benefits than other healthy foods.

Adding superfoods to your diet can help to ensure you obtain optimal nutrition as many of these foods are packed with vitamins, minerals, amino acids and often have additional health benefits. Superfoods can easily be incorporated into your diet, and are especially helpful when added to smoothies when you don't feel like eating a heavy meal.

Hemp Seeds/hearts

Hemp hearts are the edible interior part of the hemp seeds which does not contain any of the active ingredient found in its partner plant - cannabis sativa. So don't worry, you won't get high on hemp hearts.

There is a long list of health benefits that hemp hearts can offer. They are a great source of fibre and packed with vitamins. Hemp hearts contain all of the nine essential amino acids and are also a great source of vitamin E and minerals, such as phosphorus, potassium, sodium, magnesium, sulphur, calcium, iron and zinc.

Hemp seeds are nutty and sweet like pine nuts and offer a high amount of omega-3 fatty acids. Three tablespoons (30 g) of hemp hearts contain ten grams of protein — more than the amount found in a large boiled egg.

Hemp hearts can provide a topping to your dishes – sprinkle them on salads, granola or cereal, mix them into a veggie burger recipe, or blend them into smoothies.

Chia Seeds

Not only are chia seeds highly nutritious, but they may also help with inflammation due to being high in omega 3 oils.

Packed with zinc, potassium and B vitamins, they also have high amounts of magnesium and manganese. They don't have much of a flavour either, so they are great to incorporate into your diet if you just need a bit of a nutritional boost.

They are easy to include in your diet – I just throw a few spoons-full into soups or add to my morning oats. You will find many recipes online using chia seeds - in smoothies, chia jam, chocolate pudding or added to baked items.

Camu camu

Camu camu is a fruit that is native to South America and is rich in many nutrients. This fruit contains very high levels of Vitamin C as well as potassium, magnesium, manganese, copper and amino acids (serine, leucine and valine).

Camu camu is easy to take in powder form added to smoothies or sprinkled over sweet dishes.

Quinoa

Quinoa is gluten-free, high in protein and one of the few plant foods that contain sufficient amounts of all nine essential amino acids. It is also high in fibre, magnesium, B vitamins, iron, potassium, calcium, phosphorus, vitamin E and various beneficial antioxidants.

Two flavonoids that have been particularly well studied are quercetin and kaempferol and both are found in high amounts in quinoa. These important compounds have been shown to have anti-inflammatory, anti-viral, anti-cancer and anti-depressant effects in animal studies.

Quinoa can be used as a side dish in place of carbs and added to soups, curries and stews.

Maca Powder

The maca plant, is sometimes referred to as Peruvian ginseng. The main edible part of the plant is the root and it comes in several colours, ranging from white to black.

Maca root is generally dried and consumed in powder form, but it's also available in capsules and as a liquid extract. The taste of maca root powder, which some people dislike, has been described as earthy and nutty. It is often added to smoothies, oatmeal and sweet treats.

Maca root is a good source of carbs, is low in fat and contains a reasonable amount of fibre. It's also high in certain essential vitamins and minerals, such as vitamin C, copper and iron.

Maca can also be used to help reduce estrogen in your system – *more details further on.*

Bee pollen

Bee pollen is a natural mixture of flower pollen, nectar, bee secretions, enzymes, honey and wax used as a nutritional supplement. Natural health practitioners promote it as a superfood due to its nutrient-rich profile that includes tocopherol, niacin, thiamine, biotin, folic acid, polyphenols, phytosterols, enzymes, and co-enzymes.

Bee pollen is a great brain booster and is said to improve alertness and help concentration levels as well as increase general energy levels. Bee pollen is rich in the B vitamins; B1, B2 and B3 – these are essential for a healthy nervous system and powerful detoxifiers, especially to the brain.

Bee Pollen can be eaten raw or added to your favourite cereals and smoothies or mixed into yogurt. There are no set dosages for Bee Pollen but 5-10g (1-2 teaspoons) is the usual recommended daily dose.

Moringa

Moringa is a superfood which comes from the moringa tree which is loaded with nutrients including 40+ anti-oxidants, very high vitamin C levels, vitamin A, very high potassium, vitamin E, Iron (25 times more than spinach), calcium, protein (4 times more than eggs), high in B vitamins, essential minerals and amino acids.

Proposed benefits include anti-inflammatory, increases energy, detoxifying, improves wound healing, strengthens immune system, anti-depressant and improves skin health. Moringa comes as a powder and you can add it to smoothies, blend the powder into recipes like soups, dressings and pasta sauces.

Sprouted grains and seeds

Sprouts are the edible germinated seeds of beans, legumes, vegetables or grains. Sprouts deserve to be called a superfood not only because they can be grown effortlessly and inexpensively, but also because they contain exceptional amounts of vitamins and minerals, sometimes way beyond what a mature plant can offer.

When sprouting seeds, nuts, beans, and grains you obtain:

- Higher amounts of vitamins and enzymes
- Increased essential fatty acid and fibre content
- Increased bio-availability of minerals and protein

Despite their size, sprouts should never be underestimated. They are a powerhouse of nutrients. For instance, sunflower sprouts and pea shoots are known to be up to 30 times more nutritious compared to organic vegetables.

Sprout options and the nutrients they contain include:

- Alfalfa – vitamins A, B, C, D, E, F, and K
- Wheatgrass – vitamins B, C, and E
- Mung beans – protein, fibre, and vitamins C and A
- Lentil sprouts – 26 percent protein and can be eaten without cooking

Sprouting is easily done, and once germinated can be kept in the fridge in polythene bags for up to a week. Most people grow sprouts in glass jars covered with nylon mesh held in place with an elastic band around the neck. You can also buy special sprouting containers from health-shops.

As well as the great nutritional benefits of eating sprouted seeds and pulses, the other benefit is that you can feed yourself very cheaply by sprouting them yourself, and you can be confident that you are eating fresh organic food. By eating a mixture of different sprouts, you can provide your body with just about all the vital nutrients and minerals your body needs.

Time to get to the shops and buy yourself a seed sprouting kit!

There are other foods that are often included in the superfoods list include Acai berries, Goji berries and Blueberries all of which are high in nutrients. No doubt you will find other foods that are classed as superfoods each having a broad range of benefits and nutritional content.

Tip: When using smaller nuts and seeds, it is advisable to grind/mill them before adding them to your dishes or recipes in order to obtain the nutrients, otherwise they can pass though without you gaining the benefits.

How To Sprout Seeds & Pulses

The seeds and grains you can use for sprouting are cheap and readily available in supermarkets and health stores – chickpeas/garbanzos, brown lentils, mung beans, alfalfa etc. They are easy to sprout and all you have to add is fresh water. You then have easily accessible, organically grown fresh sprouts that are packed full of goodness.

Sprouting seeds instructions

- Place two handfuls of seeds or beans in the bottom of a jar or bowl and cover with plenty of water - use at least one-part seed to three parts water. Leave to soak overnight.
- Next day, pour the seeds into a sieve and rinse well with water. Be sure to remove any dead or broken seeds. If you are using glass jars then return the soaked seeds to the jar after rinsing and draining well and cover with cheesecloth secured with a rubber band and keep in a warm dark place. They can even be covered with a bag or a cloth to create darkness.
- Rinse thoroughly twice a day and be sure to drain them well or you will find they may become mouldy.
- While they are sprouting, the hulls of some seeds come off - usually while you are rinsing them. Discard the hulls as they tend to rot easily. You can do this by placing the sprouts in a big bowl of water and shaking it gently to separate the hulls from the sprouts themselves. Usually, the hulls sink to the bottom.
- After about three days, place the seeds in sunlight for several hours to develop the chlorophyll. Rinse once more in a sieve, drain well and put in a polythene bag in the refrigerator to use in salads, stir-fries etc.

There are many different seeds you can sprout, each with their own particular flavour and texture. Some sprouts, such as radish or mustard are zesty and add fire to a dish. They mix well with milder sprouts such as alfalfa or mung.

You can now buy special kits and jars to sprout your seeds. The jars have a mesh lid which makes rinsing the seeds easier. You can also buy seeds that come in selection packs which allows you to try out different seed mixes.

This is micro-gardening at its best and the reward is being able to feed yourself with fresh, nutritious organic sprouts every day.

Add 'Punch' To Your Breakfast

As we have looked at superfoods, I thought I would give you a few ideas how to add some of these to your breakfast.

Here are a few ways to add more 'punch' and healing power to your breakfast and a good way to start the day. If you are having a chia pudding, porridge or overnight oats for example, it is really easy to get some extra benefits from your breakfast by adding extra ingredients. Always aim to add some protein to your breakfast as this helps to stabilize your blood sugar levels.

For example:

- Teaspoon Bee pollen - full of vitamins, minerals and small amount of protein
- Teaspoon of MSM powder - helps with inflammation and pain
- Scoop of collagen powder - good for hair, nails, skin and scar tissue, and is a good source of protein
- Couple of teaspoons of coconut oil – healing for the gut and helps reduce Candida, and provides energy
- Scoop of protein powder - hemp is really good for providing extra nutrients and providing some extra protein
- Measure of aloe vera juice added to your smoothie - great for the gut and has lots of nutrients
- Sprinkle of sesame seeds - adds a nice texture and slightly nutty flavour, rich in nutrients - iron, manganese, calcium
- Sprinkle of hemp seeds - high in minerals and vitamins as well as protein
- Nutritional yeast - packed with B vitamins including B 12 which helps support your adrenal glands. It is also a great source of protein, manganese, iron and magnesium. Ideally you only want to sprinkle this on savoury dishes as it tastes cheesy (which is why it is added to vegan cheese recipes). You could sprinkle it on savoury muffins, or if you are OK with eggs you could have scrambled/poached egg on gluten free toast or muffin

You can mix and match some of these ideas so that you get a variety of nutritional benefits. The body can get used to certain nutrients or supplements, so switching things around will help to keep things in balance.

Green Tea Benefits

There are many health benefits to be gained by consuming green tea. One health benefit in particular which is appropriate for women with endometriosis is the ability of green tea to protect the body at a molecular level from the **toxic effects of dioxins**, and dioxins have been cited as being a possible cause of endometriosis.

Green tea also has the potential to protect from certain cancers including breast and colon cancer and can also inhibit the spread of cancers. It also lowers cytokines which are the inflammatory markers in your body thereby eliminating pain, and can also lower negative prostaglandins.

Additional health benefits of green tea include increasing the function of the liver and pancreas, protects the brain from oxidative stress, **and can help to raise serotonin and dopamine levels in the brain**. These are your feel-good neurotransmitters.

Green tea provides powerful antioxidant polyphenols (estimated as 25X the antioxidant activity of vitamin E and 100X that of vitamin C). It also promotes growth of friendly intestinal bacteria and decreases toxic bowel metabolites. Finally, another key benefit is the ability to greatly boost the immune system.

Ensure you purchase naturally decaffeinated green tea

Some green tea brands use the chemical ethyl acetate in the process of decaffeinating the tea, which can destroy most of the best antioxidants found in green tea. A double negative of more unwanted chemicals plus the health benefits of the tea being removed. Therefore, if you want to add green tea to you diet ensure to purchase naturally decaffeinated organic green tea.

Water - The Food Of Life

When it comes to regeneration and rejuvenating the body, water is the most important nutrient of all. When you become dehydrated the chemical reactions in your cells become sluggish. Also, your body cannot build new tissue effectively, toxic products build up in your blood-stream, your blood volume decreases and less oxygen and fewer nutrients are transported to your cells. Dehydration also makes you feel weak and tired and unable to concentrate.

The brain is seventy-five per cent water, this is why the quantity and quality of water you drink also affects how you feel and think. For mental clarity and emotional balance, you need plenty of water.

Drinking enough also provides us with energy; it stops us from having water-retention because the body is not in a state of panic and holding onto water all the time.

So, you can see the vital importance of water for our bodies to stay in balance. The quality of water you drink matters a lot. You can either buy quality spring water or get yourself a good quality water filter jug and use it always, changing the filter regularly. Bottled waters differ tremendously. Some of those sold in plastic containers in the super-market are nothing more than tap water which has been run through conditioning filters to remove the taste, while doing nothing to improve the quality.

For basic good health and support your immune-system, you need to be drinking around eight big glasses of water a day. Getting into the water habit will quench your thirst, improve your energy levels, improve the look of your skin, as well as stop you feeling sluggish.

Tip: Drinking a glass full of water as soon as you wake is a great way to start the day and will help to boost your energy and wake your brain. Better still, add some lemon juice and this will help to get your digestive system going.

Utensils For Cooking

Not many are aware that the implements they use when cooking can affect their health. Earthenware pots are sometimes glazed with lead or cadmium, which can be dangerous as the chemicals can leach out. White porcelain or glass containers are more suitable.

Copper, brass or aluminium pans should be avoided. Aluminium, especially, may be associated with digestive-system complaints ranging from mouth ulcers to piles. Aluminium in the system has also been associated with Alzheimer's disease. Non-stick Teflon coatings may lead to gut ulcers when they start to peel off as well as a host of other health problems.

Stainless steel pans are much safer and are more economic on power consumption if they have a copper insert sandwiched in the bottom, as this allows quick and even distribution of heat. Iron utensils are also recommended since they also distribute heat evenly for thorough cooking, and they may also add extra iron to food while cooking.

Cooking equipment

While on the topic of utensils, you may want to purchase some kitchen equipment to take the hard work out of preparing certain dishes and to be able to make some healthy juices and smoothies. As making juices has become more popular, there are many more choices of juicers to choose from and this has helped to make the prices more competitive.

Having said that, juicers can still be very expensive if you go for top of the range, but I have found the cheaper models can do a good job without breaking the bank. There are two basic types of juicer – centrifuge extraction or mastication extraction. The mastication type is better to obtain the best juice without degrading nutrients through oxidization, and they can also juice more types of foods. When looking for a juicer, read the reviews to find a juicer that is reported to be easy to clean and has proven to be robust.

Another piece of useful equipment will be a good all-round food processor/blender, which will enable you to make some of the interesting vegetarian alternative dishes like nut base pizza crusts, nut-based pastry cases for yummy sweet dishes you can find online, or blitzing up ice-cream made from frozen fruits and coconut milk – quick and easy.

Shopping List For Your Store Cupboard

This grocery shopping list comprises the main food items that are suggested to have in stock for your diet. You probably have a number of these items in your food cupboards already, so you won't be having to totally restock your cupboards.

This suggested list comprises the basics to have in constant supply. You will then be adding additional foods with your weekly shop of fresh produce of fruit, vegetables, meat, fish and other perishables.

Some of the ingredients may be different from your usual shopping list, but most of them are now easy to come by as more people are going gluten or dairy free, and you will probably find them in your supermarket.

Health food stores

Have a good look round your local health food store. Many of these stores will be selling items like - gluten/wheat free breakfast cereals, Almond milks, Rice milk, Coconut milk, healthy snacks, as well as host of grains, pulses, herbs and spices.

If you want to try out some of the ready meals in health stores just ensure to check ingredients for soy proteins, wheat powder/flour, gluten and unwanted additives. But keep your use of ready meals to a minimum because they are lower in nutritional value and of course they are always more expensive.

Ingredients For Your Food Cupboard

Dry foods

- Sweeteners - stevia, maple syrup, rice syrup, date sugar, honey (if you can guarantee to get organic honey)
- Selection of herb teas – chamomile, fennel and peppermint are all great for the digestive system
- Green Tea – caffeine free - lots of health benefits and can actually protect the body from dioxins
- Gluten free muesli and breakfast cereals of your choice
- Gluten free oats - used for porridge and used in various desserts. Oats have a great soothing effect on the inflammation of endometriosis
- Cacao powder - used in many sweet dishes and great for mixing with your morning oats
- Rice noodles - used for stir fry's and an alternative source of carbs
- Wheat/Gluten free pasta selection
- Rice - brown and basmati
- Various Gluten free flours - depending on the recipe
- All-round Gluten free flour which gives you easy flexibility
- Gluten free rice cakes or crackers - ideal for snacks with toppings like hummus and dips
- Almonds and other nuts of your choice - useful for grazing when you have the nibbles and used in dessert recipes e.g., nut-bases for cheesecakes, key lime pie etc
- Dried organic fruit selection - raisins, sultanas, dates. Used as natural sweeteners in dessert recipes.
- Dried pulses and lentils of your choice - there are loads of them and they have great flexibility of uses – add to casseroles and soups, dhal dishes, made in patties and fritters
- Chia seeds - packed full of nutrition and many flexible uses - add to soups or your breakfast cereal. Ideal to consume in the evening as they are high in the amino acid of tryptophan which is one of the calming amino acids to help you sleep.
- Seeds – sesame, sunflower, pumpkin – really great for snacking or sprinkling on dishes high nutritional value
- Lots of different herbs and spices

Liquid Foods/Other

- Olive oil - a good quality, extra virgin, cold pressed
- Avocado oil - can be used for cooking at higher temperatures than olive oil
- Nut oils, sesame oil, walnut oil
- Nut butter (try the ones available in the health store)

- Lemon juice - a good standby to have for many recipes
- Coconut milk - available in tins/cans and a thinner version in cartons
- Coconut oil - full of health benefits
- Rice wine vinegar - good for dressings
- Apple cider vinegar - has plenty of health benefits
- Tamari - the alternative to soy sauce
- Tahini - similar to peanut butter but made from ground sesame seeds
- Tins/Cans of: coconut milk, plumb tomatoes, chickpeas/ garbanzos, kidney beans
- Nut or rice milks - as an alternative to dairy milk

Adapting To A New Diet

Making changes to your diet is going to take a little while for you to adjust. You will need to stock your cupboards with a few new ingredients and safer alternatives. You may need to learn slightly different cooking skills, especially if preparing 'raw' foods for certain recipes. You will probably have to break some old ingrained habits, especially with regards to sugar and caffeine.

Do not try and do this all at once. Do a little at a time.
Maybe set yourself manageable weekly targets.

Adapting to diet changes:

Week one - change your hot drinks of tea and coffee and change over to healthy options with herb teas and try some sugar alternatives if you like your hot drinks sweetened.

Week two - change your lunch-time habit of having a wheat-based sandwich - change over to a healthy alternative, like buying an alternative to wheat bread or get some gluten free oat biscuits or rice cakes from your health store and adding some healthy dips and salad.

Week three - be brave and chuck out all those unhealthy ingredients from your cupboards and restock with safer alternatives. Start stocking up on gluten free alternatives and try out some alternatives to milk, like coconut milk or nut milk to see which ones you prefer.

Week four - start to write up meal plans, building in time-tables for your periods so you can plan what to cook in advance to get you through times when you do not feel like cooking. Build up a collection of your favourite chicken and fish dishes if you are continuing to eat animal protein.

Week five - gradually build up your new diet regime to include more meals and snacks based on an anti-inflammatory diet. Make sure you are not eating any soy or gluten – check all the labels on your foods and supplements to ensure you are not getting hidden gluten or soy.

Week six - continue building this new regime. Do not worry about lapses, you are only human. In a few weeks' time you will be able to detect what really upsets your system when you have a relapse. I think wheat and coffee will knock your system side-ways - it does for a lot of women

At around week ten - give yourself a huge treat - go for a lovely therapeutic massage if you can afford it. If you can't afford a trained masseur, then maybe a friend who has a natural touch could give you one. If you have no friends that are obliging then give yourself a DIY at-home spa day with a luxury bath with essential oils, a manicure, a natural face pack, maybe a castor oil pack and anything else that makes you feel good …. You deserve it.

Whatever you do, don't throw in the towel. The benefits will not come over night, but they will come. Believe me, many women have had huge benefits from changing their diet, with many being able to reduce their endometriosis symptoms immensely.

Your Ideal Diet

A few reminders:

- Ensure your diet excludes the inflammatory foods – red meat, dairy, sugar, gluten, soy
- Make sure your diet is balanced and interesting – you'll stick to the diet better if you enjoy your food
- I am a realist and if you are to eat any convenience foods/ready meals and sauces etc., always read the labels and do not buy foods with e-numbers and additives. You will get better quality convenience foods from health food stores – they do sell them, usually in the freezer or chill cabinet
- Avoid all foods that increase the bad prostaglandin production – these include red meat, sugar and dairy foods – these are the real baddies!!
- Eat those foods that boost your immune system
- Stay hydrated, especially drinking plenty of filtered water
- Aim to add in foods that support your liver and can aid detox
- Eat regular meals including complex carbohydrates to sustain your blood sugar levels

Eat more:

- Whole grains, (excluding wheat and rye), e.g., brown rice, millet, quinoa – this will give you extra fibre that will help to remove excess estrogens and will sustain blood sugar levels
- Ensure to get sufficient protein in your diet as protein helps to build muscle mass and also aids in the production of neurotransmitters
- Get a balance of both types of fibre – soluble and non-soluble
- Peas, beans and pulses – only if your gut can tolerate them as some cannot
- Seeds and nuts
- Sprouted seeds – increases nutritional value tremendously
- Vegetables and salads – in whatever form
- Fruit – raw, lightly cooked, pureed in puddings and smoothies
- Oily Fish - if unsure about safety of fish then eat fish purchased from organically raised fish farms
- Coconut oil and coconut milk - plenty of health benefits and recipe uses
- Foods high in omega 3 oils – fish oils, nuts and seeds
- Drink green tea to help eliminate toxins and protect your system

To wrap-up your diet changes

Be patient with yourself and the process of healing your body, and know that every healthy meal you eat is healing your digestive tract, supporting your immune-system and helping to heal your whole body.

The benefit of eating for endometriosis is that you will be eating foods that sustain and nourish you rather than having a quick fix of something that just satisfies a craving, which leaves you feeling poorly afterwards.

'Your journey to tasty, healthy and nutritional food starts here!'

For recipe ideas, when you start to dig around the internet you will find many healthy recipes which focus on using only natural healthy ingredients. Recipes ideas can be found on Pinterest as well as on websites that specialize on recipes that are gluten/wheat, dairy, soy, sugar or meat free. This means you don't have to feel as though you are going to be eating a bland and boring diet.

For example, you will find healthy alternatives for dairy and gluten free mac and cheese, dairy and sugar free desserts, gluten free baking, healthy alternatives for burgers, fritters, hash-browns, healthy sugar free ice-creams, and cheesecakes, gluten free pancakes and cookies .... the list goes on.

And when you don't feel like cooking because you are too ill or in too much pain, make sure you have some ready cooked meals in the freezer that you can fall back on. We looked at some meal ideas earlier.

Cooking in larger amounts allows you to have something tasty to eat for a few days and soups are ideal for this. Or else you can graze on some healthy snacks or make a green smoothie to provide you with the nutrients you need.

There are always options, so don't give up before you have even started. You will reap the rewards by reducing your symptoms and you will know you are working towards recovering your health.

Why Gut Health & Diet Are So Important

You are probably starting to get an idea of just how important it is to have a healthy gut. Your gut does a lot of work. It not only helps you digest food to provide nourishment to fuel your body and it is much more complex. Your gut is connected to your immune-system, your hormones, your emotional health, your neurotransmitters, protects you from viruses - which is why you need to look after your gut.

It's only in recent years that scientists are beginning to discover the vital importance of the link between diet, gut bacteria and the immune system.

One more time .... your gut is home to 80% of your immune system

Most people, including many physicians, do not realize that 80% of your immune system is located in your digestive tract, making a healthy gut a major focal point if you want to achieve optimal health. If you want to fix your health, start with your gut. Gut health literally affects your entire body.

Your Second Brain

Your gut has a nervous system that acts as a second brain. Researchers have found that the gut-brain connection plays an important part in gastrointestinal function and also relates to emotions and intuitive decision-making – your gut feeling!

Besides your brain, your gut is the only organ with its own nervous system. Your small intestine alone has as many neurons as your spinal cord. Your gut nerve cells produce 95% of your serotonin, and every type of neurotransmitter you find in your brain also exists in your gut. Your gut, in fact contains more neurotransmitters than your brain, which is why you need to nurture your gut health to support emotional health.

Your gut produces most of your neurotransmitters which are responsible for mood, sleep, motivation and energy

Neurotransmitters produced in the gut:

Serotonin - regulates sleep and appetite

Dopamine - is the feel-good chemical, plays an important role in mood, energy, attitude, motivation.

GABA - acts as your calming neurotransmitter, helping you relax and aid with sleep

Acetylcholine - for processing information and memory

You can understand then, why the gut must be in balance for your brain to be in balance. Gut-brain disturbances can show up as a wide range of disorders, including inflammatory gastro-intestinal disorders.

We have all heard of 'gut feelings', and we are all familiar how that feels – like butterflies in your stomach, or feeling nausea with anxiety.

Many issues that can disrupt your gut health

Your gut can have a hard time keeping things balanced. We looked earlier at some of the issues that can damage or upset your gut. To recap these can include:

Bad diet – eating junk food and comfort eating, especially too much sugar and inflammatory foods

Drug treatment – including anti-biotics, hormone treatment, pain medication, anti-depressants

Infections and gut imbalances - including small intestinal bacteria overgrowth (SIBO), Leaky Gut, IBS and yeast overgrowth (Candida)

Toxic overload – from household cleaners, environmental chemicals and toiletries

Stress - chronic stress alters your gut nervous system, and can create a leaky gut and changes to the normal bacteria in the gut.

Rebalancing Your Gut

- Aim to reduce your drug intake
- Ensure you eat an anti-inflammatory diet including a good daily intake of vegetables
- Replace needed enzymes and add in prebiotic foods
- Repopulate your gut with good bacteria (probiotics) to balance your gut microbiome
- To repair the gut lining include omega 3 fatty acids and zinc and refer back to supplements included in 'Supplements to heal the gut'.
- Balancing your hormones will help to rebalance your gut
- Try to reduce your stress levels to aid healing the gut

THEREFORE, YOUR GUT IS THE SEAT OF MANY EMOTIONS, YOUR IMMUNE SYSTEM AND MANY OTHER VITAL FUNCTIONS – THIS IS WHY GUT HEALTH IS SO IMPORTANT

Diet Feedback

Diet has been best treatment .....

'I have tried many different treatments to help with my endometriosis, but none of them have been of any long-lasting help. I was diagnosed with a laparoscopy 4 years ago and the doctor removed some of the implants and a few of the adhesions while operating. (I had symptoms of pain for at least 2 years before this).

I was then given hormone drug treatment to put me into a menopause. This helped for a while but the side effects were dreadful. In fact, they seem worse than my original endometriosis symptoms. I suffered severe weight gain, my skin became very greasy, I had severe trouble with sleeping, and felt really ill most of the time.

I came off the drug treatment as not only did I not want to continue, but I did not want the long-lasting side effects like bone loss. At one time I tried the BCP but again the side effects were awful. I would wake up every morning feeling really nauseous and it would last nearly all day. I tried that for 6 days and gave up.

I did not know what to do to try and deal with this disease. So, I decided to give the diet a go as I had read about it on various endometriosis boards and many of the women were saying how helpful it was. I started the diet about 5 months ago and I have never felt better. The pain I suffered for most of the time has almost gone. My pain levels with my period is about 3, on a scale of 10. I feel much healthier and suffer less bloating.

I wish I had tried the diet earlier, but I was under the illusion that medical treatment was the answer. I am now thinking of going to see a naturopath in my area and see if I can improve things even more. I really want to save - or improve - my fertility as I am still hoping and praying to have a family one day.

Girls, do give the diet a try. It is natural, safe and for me has been much better than using the dreadful drugs for treatment with all the awful side effects, hugs to you all :)' Janine

Supplements

&

Remedies

to Provide

Support

> *'If it came from a plant, eat it.*
> *If it was made in a plant, don't.'*
>
> *Michael Pollan*

Supplements – An Introduction

You often hear that you should not rely on supplements to support your health and should support your body through diet. However, as a nutritionist and health coach, this is something I feel is not always realistic when you suffer from serious illness. Supplements and herbs can help when you are really struggling and dealing with some really distressing symptoms, which can be relieved with additional help.

Also, you may not be able to obtain your nutritional needs through diet, which may be due to poor soil quality reducing the nutrients in food, or you may have trouble absorbing your nutrients while you are working to heal and healing the gut.

Aviva Romm MD who has written many women's health books and Lara Briden ND the author of 'Period Repair Manual' both recommend the use of supplements to help with endometriosis.

So why not make use of nature's bounty to obtain their healing properties. Just be sure there are no contraindications with any drugs you are currently using. It's also advised to take a rest from your supplements now and then, to give your body time to reset.

Note – getting to the root cause of your pain and other symptoms will eventually minimize your need for supplements.

Supplements are able to help with the following:
- Reducing estrogen
- Reduce bloating
- Help with pain
- Reduce scar tissue
- Help with inflammation
- Help with constipation
- Repair the gut
- Help with detoxification
- Reduce negative prostaglandins

Tips About Buying Your Supplements

Like everything you put in your body, when you are considering a supplement, you must make sure it will do you good, not harm. Many supplements contain fillers and additives which can cause further problems for your health. Here is a list of specific ingredients to avoid.

What to Avoid:

Gluten - whether you think you are gluten sensitive or not, this protein is a known inflammatory agent and can contribute to leaky gut, as well as causing an inflammatory reaction in the body and the gut.

Hidden Sugars - Sugar is known to be a cause of inflammation.

Allergens & Fillers - If you have any autoimmune disease issues, you will be sensitive to allergens. Read the labels carefully and avoid known triggers, or common inflammatory ingredients, such as corn-derived fillers.

GMO - (Genetically Modified Organisms) Ingredients – There is much controversy about the detriments of eating GMO foods or products that are derived from GMO crops. If you have an autoimmune condition, or want to decrease inflammation, it is better to avoid GMO products, whenever possible. They contain more pesticides than other plants, and there has been research showing their inbred 'pesticide' creates leaky gut.

Carrageenan - This popular vegan thickener is derived from red seaweed. However, studies indicate it can contribute to severe gastrointestinal distress and inflammation. It is found in many health supplements and products these days, so keep an eye out for this one.

Ingredients to aim for:

Vegan Friendly - Even if you are not vegan, you may prefer to stick to vegetable-based capsules and ingredients, wherever possible.

Organic Ingredients - Organic is the best option: avoiding pesticides, food irradiation, and GMO ingredients and makes choosing organic the best option.

'Free from' – many supplement manufacturers now list the 'Free from' ingredients, especially soy, gluten, additives, eggs, dairy, nuts.

About taking supplements

It is not advised to start taking lots of different supplements all at once, otherwise you will not be able to monitor the changes or benefits from any particular supplement. It is best to work with a nutritionist or natural therapist to make decisions about which supplements are best for you.

So, don't start throwing a lot of supplements into the mix in the hope of gaining relief, besides which many supplements take a while to take effect and provide results. Herbs and supplements obviously do not work the same as medication and require patience to feel the benefits.

But the advantage of using natural options as opposed to using drugs to help with your symptoms is that you can actually address the root cause, like reducing inflammation, reducing the triggers for pain, reducing estrogen and supporting the immune system.

Managing Endometriosis With Supplements

If you are taking pain-killing drugs to try and manage your symptoms there is always the risk of side-effects and eventually tolerance can build up and you have to take higher and higher doses to get any relief. However, there are certain supplements that have been found to be very effective, to not only help with pain and inflammation, but can also help reduce cysts and scar tissue.

Let's have a look at the supplements that can help with your symptoms - some of these supplements have been evaluated in research to assess their benefits for endometriosis and have been found to be very effective.

NAC

N-acetyl-cystine is a powerful supplement which can increase glutathione which is one of the most powerful detoxifiers produced in the body. It is also a great antioxidant and has helped many to reduce their symptoms of pain with endometriosis. In a 2013 study of ninety-two women in Italy, forty-seven took NAC and forty-two took a placebo. Of those who took 600 mg of NAC three times a day, **twenty-four patients cancelled their scheduled laparoscopy** due to a decrease or disappearance of endometriosis, improved pain reduction, or because they had become pregnant.

NAC is also reported to help with depression by regulating the activity of neurotransmitters (brain chemistry) especially glutamate and improving antioxidant defences in the brain. It also reduces inflammation in the brain.

Omega 3 oils – at the risk of repeating myself!

This is one supplement that should be taken by everyone – not only those with endometriosis. It helps to **reduce inflammation, reduce pain, helps to produce the good anti-inflammatory prostaglandins** and can even help with mood and protect the brain.

Omega 3 can help with mood, anxiety and depression due to its effect on calming inflammation in the brain as well as in the body. An additional benefit of supplementing omega 3 to fight brain inflammation, includes improved memory and cognitive function.

Omega 3 also helps reduce cortisol levels, which is obviously a benefit for those with high cortisol levels. Taking omega 3 in the evenings to help reduce your cortisol levels can aid with sleep, as high cortisol can stop you from sleeping.

There are several sources of omega 3 and a quality fish oil supplement is an obvious choice, as well as oily fish such as salmon, mackerel and tuna. You can also obtain high levels of omega 3 from plant foods such as chia and hemp seeds. Flax seed is another good source but unfortunately flax is also very high is phyto-estrogenic properties and many with endometriosis have problems with flax causing an increase in symptoms.

Evening Primrose Oil

This oil is commonly used to help endometriosis. **It's an anti-inflammatory and can also help with PMS** and another great benefit is that it can help **reduce bad prostaglandins** that cause pain and inflammation. According to the University of Maryland Medical Center, taking evening primrose oil helps correct estrogen imbalance. Dian Mills who wrote 'Endometriosis: A key to Healing Though Nutrition' also recommends taking evening primrose oil as part of her healing program.

Turmeric (Curcumin)

To resolve pain and inflammation turmeric is at the top of the list of supplements that can help both of these issues. Turmeric possesses **powerful anti-inflammatory properties** and one of the ways it does this is by preventing the brain from receiving signals from NF-kb, a molecule that is central to immune and cellular response. Turmeric has actually been found to have as much anti-inflammatory effect as several popular NSAIDs, including aspirin, ibuprofen, and naproxen.

Turmeric also has extremely high antioxidant value, which helps your body free itself from free radicals that are known to create inflammation and be part of autoimmune responses. Interestingly, a 2013 study published in the journal, *Phyto-therapy Research*, examined the effects of turmeric on depression in comparison to a leading anti-depressant. It was found that turmeric to be just as effective for depression as the pharmaceutic drugs, but much safer. It was also found that turmeric has positive effects on neurotransmitters like serotonin.

Turmeric can be hard to absorb, which is why is it is often combined with black pepper, as this helps to aid absorption. Another trick to increase the absorption is to take it at the same time as healthy oils and fats in your diet.

Resveratrol

Resveratrol is a plant-derived compound which is gaining interest in its ability to help treat endometriosis. It is found in many different plant species, berries, legumes and grasses, however the resveratrol that is found in grapes and red wines are found to be the best sources of this helpful compound.

The anti-inflammatory properties can help endometriosis, and it also contains certain compounds that can **help to inhibit the development of endometrial lesions**. Various studies have been done on resveratrol and the general outcome is that this compound has various benefits to help with endometriosis.

In animal models, Resveratrol treatment reduced the process of new blood vessel growth, **reduced the growth rate of endometriomas**, and reduced inflammatory markers.

Another supplement that is similar to Resveratrol is Pterostilbene, and has a very similar molecular structure and is reported to much more well absorbed following ingestion.

Serrapeptase

This supplement has had great results in **reducing scar tissue as well as reduce adhesions** and I have received a lot of good feedback from others saying how much help they have had from Serrapeptase.

It is a powerful enzyme and has really good anti-inflammatory benefits and it actually eats old scar tissue. If you have had many surgeries then you probably have scar tissue that needs resolving, and serrapeptase will help to reduce scarring and adhesions. *More details later.*

DLPA

DL-Phenylalanine is actually a substance that is made in the body and supplementing with DLPA helps to protect the body's naturally produced pain killing endorphins (the body's morphine). Increasing your endorphins can also support your immune system as well, which is a topic we cover further on regarding hormones and pain.

It takes a few days to start building up in the body before you feel the real benefits. Interestingly DLPA can help with depression – as it helps with endorphin support. Many have had success with this supplement and I personally have used it with success – much safer than taking pain meds.

Milk Thistle

This herb is excellent at supporting and detoxing your liver, and your liver is the key organ to help off-load excess estrogen from the body. Always take Milk Thistle away from meals as it can reduce your absorption of iron. (*Refer back to supplements to support the liver for more details of milk thistle*).

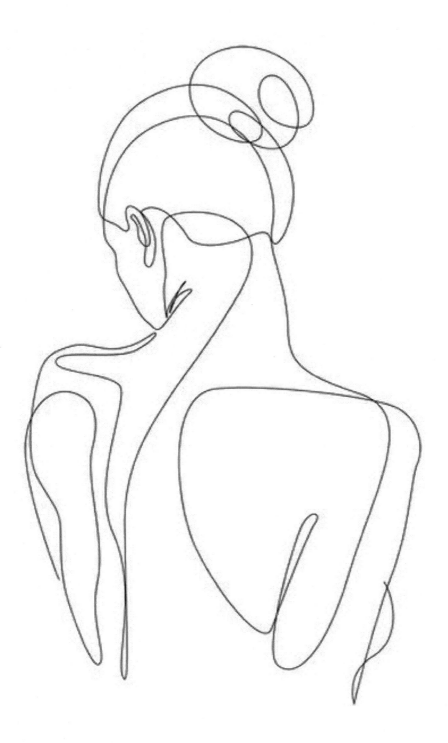

Supplements To Help Remove Estrogen

It is well known that endometriosis is fed by estrogen and many women with endometriosis have a tendency to develop estrogen dominance. It is not difficult to become estrogen dominant considering there are many chemicals in the environment that mimic estrogen and many foods contain compounds that act like estrogen called phyto-estrogens. Even the toiletries and household cleaners you use can act like estrogens which are known as xeno-estrogens.

Estrogen dominance is simply an imbalance
in the ratio of estrogen to progesterone

DIM (diindolylmethane)

DIM is one of the best-known supplements for helping to reduce estrogens. DIM supports and also improves the process of estrogen breakdown by the liver, and increases conversion of estrogen to more favourable metabolites.

One key benefit to DIM is its ability as a protective role to reduce the effects of xeno-estrogens from the environment. It may be worth trying DIM for a short while to see how it affects you, starting at a low dose and assess your reaction. Supplementing with DIM seems to upset some women causing changes in their cycle, so be mindful of any changes.

N-acetyl-cysteine (NAC)

We looked at this supplement earlier to help with endometriosis and NAC is an excellent supplement to help protect the liver and remove estrogen safely from the body. As NAC increases the level of glutathione in the liver it enhances estrogen metabolism and helps to rebalance female hormones. Taking vitamin C aids in the metabolism of NAC. Additionally, a study has shown that 1000mg of Vitamin C in addition to NAC taken every day for six months can considerably increase your progesterone production.

Maca

Peruvian Maca root is a vegetable root or tuber, related to the potato and the Mexican Wild Yam. Maca root has been used by the native Peruvians since before the time of the Incas for both its nutritional and medicinal properties. Maca root is an 'herbal adaptogen'. This means it will adapt to your body's needs, helping to naturally balance your hormones. The hormone balancing properties of maca are able to reduce estrogen levels. The recommended dose is 500mg, taken twice per day.

Some women have obtained good benefits from Maca, while for others it has upset their hormonal balance. Therefore, it is advisable to experiment and start with a low dose and see how you react.

Chaste tree berry (Vitex)

This berry supports the pituitary gland to produce progesterone and luteinizing hormone — both of which are necessary for your body to ovulate, for regular menstrual cycles and to avoid symptoms of hormonal imbalance. Maintaining a healthy ratio of progesterone to estrogen is important for female reproductive function, and vitex acts to regulate levels, which can support fertility and menstruation.

Vitamin B6

An excess of estrogen can be re-balanced by taking B6 which can help to boost your natural progesterone production. B6 supports the development of the corpus luteum (the corpus luteum is a temporary endocrine gland the female body produces after ovulation during the second half of the menstrual cycle and is involved in the production of progesterone).

B6 also specifically works with liver enzymes to remove excess estrogen from the body and boosts the immune system to prevent autoimmune response.

Serrapeptase Benefits For Endometriosis

As we are looking at specific supplements to help with your symptoms, this one stands out for having great success to help reduce scar tissue and adhesions.

What is Serrapeptase?

Serrapeptase is a proteolytic enzyme which is found in silkworms. The silkworm uses it to dissolve the cocoon when the moth is ready to come out. Serrapeptase is used for many painful conditions as it has the ability to reduce inflammation, it helps to dissolve old scar tissue and reduce adhesions and cysts. One of the main actions it has is to dissolve fibrin, and scar tissue is made up of fibrin.

Fibrin and scar tissue

Fibrin is produced in the body as a chemical product to help stop bleeding and is used as part of the healing process following injury or surgery. It has a useful purpose initially in the role of healing, however if the area in question is slow to heal, an excess of fibrin will appear as clumps of scar tissue in the site of the wound, injury or at a surgical site.

Once this happens, an acute condition becomes chronic. For women with endometriosis this action can cause a severe excess of fibrin in the body caused by bleeding implants, scar tissue and post-operative scarring as well.

To help with scar tissue and endometriosis, Serrapeptase basically digests non-living tissue, blood clots, cysts, arterial plaque and inflammation in all forms. Additionally, it helps improve the immune response, helps with pain and assists with speeding the healing process.

How to take Serrapeptase

Serrapeptase needs to be taken on an empty stomach at least 45 minutes before eating or two hours after eating.

Serrapeptase is easily destroyed and deactivated by your stomach acid before it has a chance to reach your intestines to be absorbed. For this reason, supplements of Serrapeptase should be enteric-coated, which prevents them from being dissolved in the stomach and allows for release in the intestine.

Serrapeptase is available in various dosages and it is advised to start low and build up your dosage. A good starting dose is 80,000iu per dose taken twice a day. Some Serrapeptase supplements are as high as 250,000iu but it is not advisable to start on such a high dose with a supplement you have not taken before. It is safer to see what your reaction is to a lower dose first and then work your way up.

Possible serrapeptase side effects

Some women experience increased bleeding with their period due to blood thinning effects, so maybe start at a low dose and monitor your reaction, and do not take with other blood thinning supplements including turmeric and garlic.

- Advised to stop serrapeptase 2 weeks before surgery as it may increase risk of bleeding
- Serrapeptase may cause blood thinning so it is advised not to take with turmeric, fish oil, gingko biloba, and vitamin E

Feedback for serrapeptase

It really helps to read feedback from others who have used a product before you rush out to buy it. These feedback comments have been sent to me at endo-resolved and I have also had great success using this supplement when working with women with endometriosis.

'This product is an excellent anti-inflammatory. It's the only product (together with a healthy diet) that has kept my endometriosis pain and symptoms under control. I have been taking this for 6 months now and my endometrioma cyst has decreased in nearly 1cm! It has also improved my digestion; I hardly ever have stomach pain now.'

'I have now used Serrapeptase for over 6 months and I had an internal scan to check if my Endometriosis has come back on my ovaries after over 1 year of surgery. I am about to start IVF treatment and to our happy surprise no Endometriosis or scarring has been found. Everything is looking good. We are so happy that I have used this as it has not only helped enormously with keeping my pain away but also kept the Endometriosis away!! This is a miracle enzyme and I always recommend this product to my friends and family or anyone who could benefit from it. Thank you'

'Started taking these for my endometriosis pain and it has changed my life. Went from daily pain and swelling to the odd twinge maybe once a week if that. Haven't experienced any side effects. Works wonders for me and I will continue to take these.'

MSM – For Pain And Inflammation

Sulphur (Methyl Sulphonyl Methane - MSM) is a dietary supplement that can help to reduce pain and inflammation of endometriosis. It can also help soften scar tissue, which makes it helpful for post-surgery scars and may also help reduce adhesions. This is one supplement I used daily myself for my endometriosis and I still use it today to help with old horse-riding injuries.

MSM is a form of organic sulphur that is stored in every cell of our bodies. The body uses sulphur continuously to create new cells; without it the body can produce weak and dysfunctional cells.

We are supposed to get sulphur from our food but even washing food can remove the sulphur we need, and processing food certainly will. Sulphur is the third most abundant substance in our bodies.

MSM is available as a supplement in a variety of forms. I have found the cheapest to be a loose powder which I mix with orange juice, and take first thing in the morning. You can also mix it with your morning smoothie or your breakfast oats.

Feedback for using MSM

'I recently read about MSM on your website. Having gone through Hell!!!! I tried it and 3 weeks later I have had no pain!!!! It is unbelievable!! I have no pain with my periods and my endo flares are just about a thing of the past. I add the powder to my morning smoothie every day now. Thank you very much!!!!! Candy

That feedback was short and to the point, and I always recommend MSM to help with endometriosis pain and inflammation, and any other conditions that cause similar symptoms.

Vitamin D & Endometriosis

Recent studies have shown that women with endometriosis tend to have lower Vitamin D levels. Long term Vitamin D deficiencies have been linked to a weakened immune system and to chronic inflammation.

Studies have noted that low levels of vitamin D have also been connected to the severity of endometriosis and to those who had the largest ovarian cysts. While further research is needed, it appears that Vitamin D deficiency could play a key role with endometriosis and could be connected to disease severity.

Vitamin D deficiency is related to chronic pain because it plays a vital role with your nervous system

The best source of Vitamin D is direct sunlight on the skin with 10,000 to 20,000 IU of Vitamin D being produced in 30 minutes with whole-body exposure to sunlight. In the winter months with very low levels of sunlight, you are obviously not going to be able to get any serious levels of Vitamin D, so it's important, especially during this time to supplement.

You can easily get your vitamin D levels checked with a simple blood test which your doctor can do or you can order a test yourself from on-line labs.

Vitamin D & Hormones

There is a connection between vitamin D and important hormones, such as dopamine and serotonin, which can regulate your mood. This evidence is in part derived from an animal-based trial where it was found that vitamin D supplementation was capable of boosting dopamine levels in vitamin D deficient rats.

There is also evidence to suggest that vitamin D could be capable of influencing several different hormones in the body, from your thyroid hormones to sex hormones like estrogen and progesterone. (*More on this later*).

Foods high in vitamin D

Vitamin D is oil soluble, which means you need to eat fat to absorb it better. Foods high in vitamin D include:

- Salmon, Tuna, Sardines, Mackerel, Trout, Cod liver oil
- It is also found in fortified foods like cereals, orange juice and certain milk products

Vitamin D is also available as a dietary supplement, either alone or combined with other nutrients. Calcium supplements, for example, typically include vitamin D.

Whether vitamin D levels relate to the severity of endometriosis or not, having optimal levels of this vital vitamin will be of benefit to your health. As mentioned above, having low vitamin D can cause pain, make inflammation worse and have a detrimental effect on your immune system.

If you are going to supplement with Vitamin D, it is critical that you add a Vitamin K2 supplement at the same time. Vitamin D and K2 work with one another to maintain control over calcium levels in the body. Vitamin D controls the absorption of calcium into the blood, whereas Vitamin K2 controls where calcium goes in your body.

Multiple Benefits Of Magnesium

Magnesium is needed for every function in the body. However, it is easy to become deplete in this vital nutrient for various reasons.

Magnesium has a number of benefits to help endometriosis, depending on which type of magnesium is used. It can help with muscle pain, insomnia, bowel problems, provide a calming effect, support brain function and is involved in many biochemical processes in the body. Magnesium makes muscles work properly, allowing for correct muscle contraction and relaxation in combination with maintaining correct calcium levels.

How do we become deplete in magnesium?

We can easily loose vital magnesium levels through:

Drug intake (toxic chemicals), low levels of digestive enzymes, stress, sugar intake, alcohol, and diuretics.

Magnesium helps different functions:

Citrate – Bowel Problems

This form is inexpensive and easily absorbed. This is helpful as a constipation aid and it has a very fast absorption rate.

Glycinate – Relaxing

This form is very calming and good to take in the evening for sleep. This form is very good for leaky gut, nerve pain, chronic pain, and it is very bio-available

Malate – Energy Fuel

This is great for muscle pain if you are suffering from fatigue or have fibromyalgia. It has malic acid which is a natural fruit acid and can aid digestion.

Sulphate – Epsom Salts

This form soothes muscles and is commonly referred to as Epsom salts. Added to your bath water to aid relaxation as well as soothes muscle pain.

Taurate – Cardiovascular Health

This has been described as the best choice for cardiovascular issues as it prevents arrhythmias and heart attacks. It stabilises nerve cells, contracts heart muscles and improves blood pressure.

L-Threonate – Brain Function

This version works great for mental sharpness and cognitive health. This benefits anyone suffering from depression, anxiety, PTSD.

As well as supplementing you can increase your magnesium intake with certain foods. The best sources of magnesium are found in the following:

Spinach, Chard, Pumpkin Seeds, Avocado, Banana, Dark Chocolate, Quinoa, Almonds, Black Beans, Cashews, Figs, Yogurt, and Bananas.

Women with endometriosis are often lacking in magnesium due to estrogen dominance. During menstruation, women's magnesium levels can be reduced by up to 50%, further depleting their supply. As magnesium helps to reduce cramping, having optimal levels in your body can help reduce endometriosis pain.

Magnesium Spray for pain relief

Magnesium is great for pain relief and when you apply directly to your skin, it will soak in and help relieve pain directly where it is needed. You can purchase magnesium sprays, but they can be expensive. You can easily make your own pain relief magnesium spray at home with very few ingredients, and you will know there are NO added ingredients.

Shopping list:

- Magnesium chloride flakes – from your local pharmacy or health websites
- Distilled water

You need:

- Half cup magnesium flakes
- Half cup distilled water
- Spray bottle
- Pain relied essential oils of choice

To make:

- Boil the distilled water and pour it on the magnesium flakes.
- Stir vigorously until the flakes are completely dissolved.
- Add a few drops of essential oils of choice
- After the water cools down, transfer the mixture to a spray bottle.

Notes:

Will keep for up to six months.

This blend will cost about 1/10th the cost of purchasing ready-made magnesium oil and the benefit is you can add other pain-relieving ingredients.

Essential oils to add for pain relief include:

Chamomile, peppermint (anti-spasmodic), lavender (can help menstrual cramps), eucalyptus (great for nerve related pain), rosemary (analgesic and anti-inflammatory), copaiba (excellent for pain relief).

Yarrow Benefits For Endometriosis

Yarrow tea has traditionally been used to ease menstrual cramps. It helps by relaxing smooth muscles in your uterus. It's a good idea to start drinking this tea a couple of days before your periods begin - 2 cups of tea a day should help.

Yarrow also has a long-established use as a sleeping aid. Yarrow extract has sedative as well as anti-anxiety effects. Yarrow contains a mild hypnotic ingredient called thujone, which has a similar effect to that of marijuana which provides a calming effect. A cup of yarrow tea in the evening will help you relax and assist with sleep.

Another common problem that a cup of yarrow tea can help is indigestion. According to research, compounds found in yarrow can increase bile flow and promote pancreatic juices to flow, and bile helps break down fat and improve digestion. If your liver is sluggish then yarrow will help improve its function and protect the liver from damage.

Yarrow can be used in the following ways:

Herbal tea, capsules, tincture, essential oil

Start with yarrow tea rather than capsules at first to see how you react to it, drinking 2 cups a day between meals. One great benefit of yarrow essential oil is to help with menstrual cramps due to being anti-inflammatory and has anti-spasmodic properties on the muscles, and mixed with a carrier oil can be massaged over your abdomen.

Precautions:

Yarrow tea should only be consumed for up to 7-10 days in succession, and then skipped for a few days. Yarrow tea should not be consumed by pregnant women as it relaxes the smooth muscles of the uterus and may induce miscarriage. *Yarrow may also cause photo-sensitivity*

Also, yarrow should not be used if you are on a prescription sedative or anxiety medication or if you are taking medication for high blood pressure or heart disease. Yarrow should not be taken when using Tylenol as it has an adverse effect on the liver.

Natural Remedies To Support Your System

To help you support your system naturally when trying to cope with endometriosis there are various gentle natural remedies you can use. I have provided this list of natural everyday remedies, vitamins and supplements you can use to support your body.

You can view this list more as a First Aid/Quick reference list to dip into to give you extra support when you feel the need.

Stress relief

Trying to cope with endometriosis on a daily basis can cause a lot of stress and anxiety. There a few gentle natural remedies you can try to help reduce your stress levels and calm your system.

- Niacin – small dose after meals – calms nerves/anxiety. Niacin can cause flushing in many and using niacinamide can overcome this issue
- Theanine – calming amino acid, also good before bed to calm the mind
- Aromatherapy – certain oils are very calming and can help calm the central nervous system – Chamomile, Lavender, Vetiver, Ylang ylang, Valerian, Jasmin, Frankincense (good for pain too)
- CBD oil – this oil is really gaining popularity to help with stress and anxiety. A couple of drops under the tongue a few times a day can help

Muscle support

Endometriosis causes a lot of muscle pain, not only in the abdomen, but other muscles can be affected. Here a few ideas that can help, including supplements, herbal teas and other natural remedies.

- Chamomile - Muscle pain and soreness – taken as a tea or used externally as an essential oil
- Tart Cherries - muscle relaxer, anti-inflammatory, & anti-oxidant – can be found in capsules or juice. Good to use in the evening as it helps to increase natural melatonin production
- Peppermint - Muscles relaxer, backaches, leg pain, & tension headaches – can be taken as a tea or used externally as an essential oil
- Cayenne Pepper - Reduce muscle pain, stiffness, & inflammation. Helps with palpitations – can be found as a tincture used in water or capsules
- Epsom Salt Bath - Relaxes the nervous system, removes toxins, & helps with pain and inflammation.
- Arnica – Homeopathic cream - Anti-inflammatory & improves blood circulation.
- Lavender - Reduces pain, swelling & inflammation – used externally as an essential oil
- Raspberry Leaf - Muscle pain & cramps – commonly used as a tea
- Magnesium oil - Topical application for muscle pain & cramps.

Depression and brain health

It stands to reason that endometriosis will cause a huge amount of mental stress, depression and anxiety. There are certain nutrients that can help to support mental health:

- Vitamin D - Mental health, Immune boosting, scar healing, bones. This vitamin (hormone) is also noted to help with endometriosis as mentioned earlier
- Lithium Orotate - Mood Stabilizer. OTC supplement (not prescription med). Lithium orotate can aid in the absorption of B12
- Vitamin B-6 - Neurological Health
- Magnesium – Calming – use magnesium glycinate for calming effects
- Fish oil - Depression
- SAMe (S-adenosyl-L-methionine) – for depression, SAMe is found naturally in the body – also supports glutathione process in the liver, which protects the liver
- Probiotics – certain probiotics are responsible for the production of neurotransmitters, which are made in the gut

Energy (or lack of!)

When we suffer a serious illness, it seems to really sap energy levels. This can happen as a natural mechanism of the body to ensure you do not over-exert yourself and stress your body, so the body is made to slow down as part of the natural healing/survival mechanism. As well as ensuring you have a balanced diet and provide all the nutrients you need to support your body you can use certain nutrients to help with energy levels.

- Pantothenic Acid - (Vitamin B-5) aids generation of energy from fat, carbohydrates and proteins. Supports adrenal gland function
- Eleuthero root – Can help chronic fatigue syndrome
- D-ribose – utilised for energy production and is often suggested for CFS
- B vitamins – the b vitamins are well known for providing energy. They also support the adrenal glands, support the nervous system and are involved in hormone production. Bee pollen is a good natural way to obtain the B vitamin complex.
- Ginseng – is well known to help with energy but some people cannot tolerate it and find it too stimulating – try a small dose and see how it affects you.
- Iron – make sure you sustain your iron levels. Ensure to take iron supplements if your doctor has prescribed them and add iron rich foods to your diet.

Low Dose Naltrexone For Endometriosis

Alternative treatment for endometriosis and auto-immune diseases

Low dose naltrexone (LDN) is an interesting compound and holds promise as an alternative treatment for endometriosis and infertility.

Low dose naltrexone is used to treat various auto-immune diseases and certain cancers with great success. Many women with endometriosis also suffer from various auto-immune diseases, therefore low dose naltrexone is gaining interest as an option for the treatment of endometriosis along with other related health issues.

Naltrexone is a type of drug called an "opiate antagonist", meaning it blocks opioid receptors. Opioid receptors are related to pain, pleasure and endorphins. Taken in low doses LDN blocks opioid receptors only for a couple of hours. During this brief time, a 'rebound effect' occurs in which there is an increased production and utilisation of endorphins and opioid receptors.

Put simply, low-dose naltrexone is blocking the cells and pathways that play a role in inflammation and consequently pain. Also, low-dose naltrexone may be able to restore endorphin production in people who suffer from ongoing fatigue, depression and anxiety.

LDN has had good results for those with cancer, neuro-degenerative conditions, autoimmune conditions, under-active thyroid, Multiple Sclerosis and many other auto-immune disorders.

In an interview with Dr. Phil Boyle Director of the NaPro Fertility Care Clinic in Dublin he discusses the benefits that can be found using LDN for infertility, auto-immune diseases and endometriosis.

'By using LDN in women who have endometriosis, we've observed a lower incidence of miscarriage and better, healthier pregnancies for women who continue using it during pregnancy. So that's the immediate reason for using LDN. But there may be an even greater impact in the form of positively affecting the health of future generations of women as well.'

How LDN can help women with endometriosis

It is well known that endometriosis is related to imbalances in your hormones but one aspect that is often overlooked is that it is also strongly linked to the immune system. Endometriosis has been shown to have similarities with various other autoimmune diseases by also presenting with elevation in inflammatory markers, cell-mediated abnormalities, raised anti-bodies and elevation of other blood markers. The use of LDN has been found to address some of these issues by rebalancing hormones as well as the immune system.

Side effects

There may be some sleep disturbance at first but this soon wears off. Sometimes headaches and vivid dreams can occur, but these side effects will also decrease with time. If sleep disturbances occur then taking the medication in the morning can resolve the problem.

Note* *You cannot mix low dose naltrexone with opioid drugs like codeine or morphine. Both codeine and morphine are opioids and if you mix Naltrexone with either of these medications, you may become sick and suffer vomiting.*

Extract of a story of success using Low Dose Naltrexone

'I believe that I had endometriosis since my first period at 12 and possibly before. It took about 10 years before getting diagnosed. And even after my diagnosis I had enough of not being taken seriously and being treated like a hypochondriac and drug seeker.

Five months before I consider myself cured, I stared taking (LDN) Low dose naltrexone which really helped with general pain relief, depression, ME and fibromyalgia. It was challenging to get a prescription.

LDN is a medication that works with your body's immune system through its interactions with your body's endorphins. Endorphins play a role in pain relief, immune system regulation, growth of cells and angiogenesis (the growth of blood vessels that feed a tumour). It is also sometimes used to improve fertility in endometriosis patients.

Now when I have my period, I no longer need to take any pain killers (not that they ever worked), and I take LDN and NAC supplements for my rosacea. It took about 2 months before I could no longer feel the adhesion that once prevented me from exercising and caused me intense pain.

I stopped being so strict with the paleo diet and stick to a more normal gluten free organic diet with no issues and diet changes have helped to keep the pain in check, especially stopping gluten.

Don't let anyone tell you that you have to live with an illness for the rest of your life when there is hope, and there are people with incurable conditions who have found healing!

The moment you are ready to quit is usually the moment right before the miracle happens!'

Conditions that may respond to LDN Therapy

Inflammatory states

Autoimmune conditions – multiple sclerosis, Lupus, rheumatoid arthritis etc. GI inflammatory bowel disease – Crohn's disease, ulcerative colitis & IBS Lung - COPD, asthma, Cancer – many different cancers respond well to LDN

Hormone dysfunctions

Thyroid - hyper & hypo-thyroid states, endometriosis, PMS, PCOD, infertility

Managing Pain

&

Supporting

Your

Immune-System

> *'The mind and body are not separate. what affects one, affects the other.'*
>
> *Anonymous*

What Causes Your Pain?

This is a very loaded question and no doubt you will often ask 'What causes all this pain?' The process of suffering pain involves many complex chemical pathways and often the pain of endometriosis has more than one cause.

A lot of the pain you feel is actually due to inflammation which is a natural bodily reaction to injury or damage to any tissue in the body.

The damaged sites, adhesions and cysts will trigger a reaction in the body that sets off the inflammatory reaction and blood vessels will dilate to increase blood flow to the area. The cells in connective tissue release histamines (increasing blood supply to a damaged site) and also release prostaglandins which cause inflammation as well as the sensation of pain.

The other obvious and common type of pain is caused by your muscles when they go into spasm – e.g., when you have menstrual cramps, and you feel these cramps through pain messenger signals sent through the body to the brain.

Some of the causes of pain include:

- A major increase in inflammatory chemicals (cytokines).
- Cyclical bleeding from endometriosis growths (endometrial implants).
- Development of scar tissue/adhesions - multiple adhesions can cause the reproductive organs to become misshapen and glued together
- Scar tissue that develops after surgery, which can then develop into adhesions
- Irritation of the pelvic floor nerves or other nerves - the pelvis has the greatest concentration of nerve fibres in the body.

Pain & endometrial implants

Endometriosis pain may be due to inflammation around the implants. The immune system will then be triggered into action and a chemical chain reaction begins with lymphokines, interleukins and inter- ferons. These white blood cells then pour into the damaged site with the aim to protect it and allow the body to heal the damage.

These cells build a protective layer around the problem which causes it to be inflamed. This in turn can put pressure on nearby nerve endings which will stimulate more pain.

Hormones and pain

Hormones also play an important role in processing or managing pain. Sleep disturbances can be caused by hormonal imbalance, often due to an imbalance between estrogen and progesterone. In turn, research has found that a lack of sleep is known to cause increased levels of pain.

The same research also found that after a sleepless night, activity in the brain where pain signals are received – increase by a whopping 126 percent. The end result of losing sleep is that you suffer more pain. We look at ways to improve your sleep further on, and reducing your pain levels will obviously help improve your chances of getting a good night's sleep.

Hormones that affect pain

Endorphins – these hormones play an important role regarding pain and the immune-system. Endorphins are hormones produced by the central nervous system and the pituitary gland. We have already looked at the role of endorphins in relation to pain in the topic of Low Dose Naltrexone.

Endorphins are the feel-good chemicals and our bodies also release this hormone during extreme pain (strange as that may sound). Endorphins interact with the receptors in your brain that reduce your perception of pain. Endorphins also trigger a positive feeling in the body, similar to that of morphine. Additionally, it has recently been found that endorphins play a role in the immune system.

Vitamin D - Low Vitamin D levels increase inflammation and pain. Vitamin D is actually a hormone. In one controlled study, people with vitamin D deficiency were nearly twice as likely to experience bone pain compared to those with optimal levels. Every tissue in our bodies has vitamin D receptors, including all bones, muscles, immune cells, and brain cells. We have already touched on vitamin D with regards to development of endometriosis, and many in the West can become deplete in this vital hormone.

Cortisol - One of the primary roles of cortisol in the body is to reduce inflammation and control your body's immune response. Over time constant stress can deplete your adrenal glands and your adrenals start to produce less cortisol. This can allow an inflammatory process within your body to be left unchecked and lead to swelling, pain and tissue damage.

Estrogen/Progesterone - an imbalance of estrogen to progesterone can increase pain and inflammation. Artificially elevated levels of estrogen, like those caused by hormone replacement therapy and oral contraception are strongly linked to joint pain. Fortunately, most women with endometriosis who use BCP treatment to calm endometriosis tend to be put on drugs which are low in estrogen.

Thyroid Levels – as well as energy production, thyroid hormones modulate muscle and nerve action. Having low thyroid levels (hypothyroidism) can lead to muscle pain and joint pain as well as a host of other symptoms.

DHEA - this is another hormone that is produced mainly by the adrenal glands. Low DHEA can cause a wide variety of symptoms including fatigue, depression, joint pain, and a host of other issues. DHEA levels can be checked with a comprehensive adrenal cortisol saliva test (*details further on*).

To sum up causes of pain

- Chemical reactions caused by damage tissue
- Immune system response
- Pressure in nerve endings
- Endometrial implants and adhesions
- Scar tissue – from past operations
- Muscle pain and spasms with menstruation
- Pain with ovulation
- Inflamed damaged tissue caused by implants
- Hormone imbalances

A few tips to help reduce your levels of pain

- Reduce inflammation through diet and increasing anti-inflammatory foods
- Ensure you are not eating trigger foods – we are all different and you need to keep a note of your own particular trigger foods
- Remove foods that promote negative prostaglandins responsible for increasing pain, which we have covered already
- Use supplements that can help to reduce inflammation and pain i.e. MSM, DLPA, CBD, Turmeric, Omega 3 oil
- Use supplements that can reduce scar tissue build up like serrapeptase and digestive enzymes

Additionally, getting some hormone tests done will also help to assess whether you are suffering pain due to hormone imbalances. I keep saying this, but hormones are very powerful and when they are out of whack you can feel really off, especially if your thyroid or cortisol levels are low – we look at thyroid and adrenal gland health further on, as well as the need for hormone testing.

Let's see how we can reduce your pain with natural remedies

Natural Pain Relief

This list of natural remedies for pain relief includes some tried and tested solutions, some of which you may be familiar with. We have already touched on a couple of remedies that can help with pain and here are a few more natural remedies that can help.

Massage - Massage can help to relieve muscle pain and tissue injury. You can do a gentle massage of your abdomen and use some essential oils that help with pain and inflammation. For muscle pain try oils of copaiba, yarrow, sage, rosemary or thyme.

Epsom salt baths - Soaking in an Epsom salts bath can really help to relax muscles and in turn help to relieve pain. You can also add a few relaxing essential oils at the same time – great to help you calm down and relax before bed.

Heat pads or hot water bottle - Using heat on the abdomen is a good way to help relax your muscles which can help to relieve your pain. You can purchase different types of heat pads these days as well as wheat bags which are heated in the microwave. Heat pads are also helpful for the low back pain that is so common with endometriosis. Be careful not to use heat pads that are too hot as they can cause skin scarring if use for too long or too hot.

TENS unit - Many have success using a TENS machine which basically sends small electric pulses to the skin where the self-adhesive pads are applied and this desensitises the nerves from feeling pain.

Castor oil packs - Castor oil packs have many health benefits – they can help with endo belly, ease cramping, calms the central nervous system, reduce inflammation, support digestion and when placed over the liver can help with detox. (*A topic covered in more detail further on*).

Acupuncture - This is a very good remedy not only for pain for other health issues which has been covered in the natural therapies section. Acupuncture is well known to have been used during surgery to relieve pain. It is said to work partly by stimulating the release on endorphins and can also help with anxiety and depression.

Menastil - This is a product that has been produced to specifically help with menstrual pain which is applied topically over the abdomen. It works by inhibiting the pain signals that travel from one nerve to another. I have had feedback from some saying they have found it helpful.

DLPA - This supplement has been covered earlier but worth a reminder ….

DL-Phenylealanine (DLPA) does not actually block the symptoms. It works instead by protecting the body's naturally produced pain killing endorphins (the body's morphine), effectively extending their life span in the nervous system. It slows the activity of "enzyme chewing" enzymes which destroy endorphins thereby giving them more time to act on areas of pain.

It is also a powerful antidepressant and in clinical studies has been proven to be as effective as commonly prescribed antidepressant drugs - without the side effects. DLPA can also relieve symptoms of PMS and has had great success in dealing with the pain of endometriosis.

Meditation - Research now shows that the use of meditation can be successful to help manage and reduce pain. MRI's show the brain of a person meditating has a significant decrease in pain reception. Meditation can actually change the way the mind perceives pain so that it's more bearable. It is a natural and effective way to ease physical pain.

In fact, meditation can help induce the body's natural opioid system, and mediation can also help reduce anxiety and stress. There are numerous videos on YouTube that provide guided meditations specifically to help with pain relief. You may have to practise to get used to meditating, but the more you do it, the easier it will get.

CBD Oil For Pain Relief

CBD oil is used with success by many with endometriosis for pain and insomnia. As well as helping with pain, CBD oil can also help with inflammation, is reported to help with cancer, can aid with anxiety and can even help relieve certain types of seizures and epilepsy.

Researchers compiled the results of multiple reviews, covering dozens of trials and studies into the use of CBD oil for pain. Their research concluded that there is substantial evidence that CBD is an effective treatment for chronic pain.

The fascinating thing about CBD therapy is that the body actually has cannabinoid receptors, which form part of the endocannabinoid system – *who would have thought!*

The body produces two receptors:

CB1 receptors are present throughout the body, particularly in the brain. They co-ordinate movement, pain, emotion, mood, thinking, appetite, memories, and other functions.

CB2 receptors are more common in the immune system. They affect inflammation and pain.

CBD stimulates the receptors so that the body produces its own cannabinoids, known as endocannabinoids.

What Is the Endocannabinoid System?

Breaking down the word 'endocannabinoid', 'cannabinoid' comes from 'cannabis,' and 'endo' is short for 'endogenous,' which means that it is produced naturally inside of your body. So 'endocannabinoid' simply means cannabis-like substances that naturally occur inside the body.

Purchasing CBD oil

As well as oil, CBD can also be purchased as bath bombs to provide a relaxing bath, lotions to apply direct to areas of pain, vaping oil for smoking and even sold as suppositories which can be used in the rectum or inserted in the vagina to help with pelvic pain.

The oil comes in many different strengths and it is recommended to start at a low dose and work up in strength. You need to take care where you purchase your oil, as there are many products on the market as the oil is gaining in popularity, and some oils can be very poor in quality. It is often advised to ask for recommendations, or try to find online reviews to help you decide which is the best product.

CBD oil suppositories

CBD suppositories are very effective for pelvic pain; however, they can be very expensive. In fact, I was stunned at the price, at $7/£5 for a single suppository, so I decided to make my own. You can easily make your own suppositories by purchasing suppository moulds. I found that using coconut oil mixed with CBD oil is an easy method to make your own suppositories – and so much cheaper. You can buy strips of plastic suppository moulds from various sources online as well as your local chemist.

To make a dozen CBD suppositories

1. Melt a couple of tablespoons of coconut oil in a glass bowl placed in hot water (coconut oil has a very low melt point, so you don't need to heat it on the stove)
2. Add sufficient CBD oil to allow for 2 drops for each suppository and mix with the coconut oil.
3. Pour the mixture into the suppository moulds, you may find a cheap plastic syringe makes this job easier.
4. You can buy some moulds that come with a stand to hold them upright while they set. Or you can devise a way to support cheaper moulds upright while the oil sets. I just cut a strip of plastic suppository moulds of a required length which can that be wedged inside a plastic food container without falling over.
5. Put the filled moulds in the fridge to set. Once the oil has hardened the suppositories are then ready to use. Keep them in the fridge so they stay hard and only take them out when you want to use one.

You can use CBD suppositories vaginally or rectally and both will help to provide the pain-relieving benefits and is a quick way for your body to absorb the oil. Using them rectally can help with bowel inflammation, irritable bowel and I have read reviews of helping with ulcerative colitis. They are also a great way to obtain CBD oil benefits for those who really do not like the taste or it upsets their stomach when taken orally.

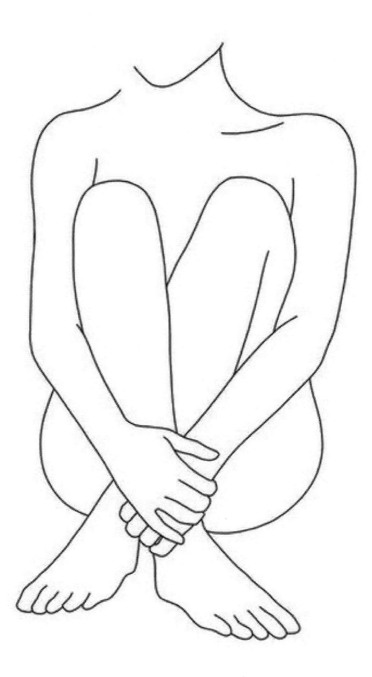

Tips For Managing Your Period Pain

Coping with period pains for many women can seem relentless, but is much worse when you have endometriosis. Quite often it means relying on heavy-duty pain medications, but there are other natural self-help remedies you can use to help manage your pain.

If you remember the subject we covered earlier about prostaglandins, diet and pain – the advice there gives you some tips of how we can reduce our pain through diet changes, and this includes your period pain.

Once you start managing your endometriosis more naturally, especially with regard to your diet, you may be surprised how much improvement you see in your period pain.

Here are some self-help measures to help ease period pain:

You may be using some of these already, but for those who need a few extra tips …

- Hot baths with essential oils and Epsom salts
- CBD oil or balm applied over pelvic area
- TENS unit – helpful for general pelvic pain and back pain
- Castor oil packs – applied over your abdomen
- DLPA supplement – taken twice a day
- Cramp Bark tea
- Ginger tea or ginger powder - has been shown to be as effective as ibuprofen and mefenamic in reducing period pain
- Ensure you have sufficient magnesium and you can also use a magnesium spray, sprayed over the pelvic region
- Copaiba oil massaged over your abdomen
- Ensure you are not eating foods that increase prostaglandins

Make sure you are eating regularly to sustain your blood sugars and don't be tempted to eat sweet sugary snacks, as sugar is very inflammatory and will make you feel worse. Buy in a supply of healthy snacks to graze on, and the good news is that dark chocolate is actually good for you – just make sure its low in sugar.

Help for heavy periods

Tranexamic acid - your doctor may prescribe this medication if you have very heavy periods. Tranexamic acid helps your blood to clot, which reduces bleeding. As with any pharma drug there can be side effects and this can include nausea, dizziness, skin rash, and even depression is noted as a side-effect.

Raspberry leaf tea - as a safe herbal option, traditionally raspberry leaf has been used to relieve painful menstruation. Raspberry tea suppresses menstrual flow by constricting body tissues, and can also be useful in reducing menstrual cramps.

Nettle leaf is another herb to consider using during menstruation as it contains vitamin K which promotes blood clotting, its rich in iron, supports liver health and can help reduce inflammation.

Herbal tea recipe for heavy periods

- ½ ounce red raspberry leaf
- ½ ounce stinging nettle leaf
- 1 quart mason jar

Instructions:

Place the herbs into the mason jar and fill the jar with boiled water. Stir to make sure the herbs are fully covered with the water. Seal the jar and allow it to sit for at least 4 hours or overnight. Sweeten with honey if desired and drink within 24 hours.

You can drink this blend daily or every other day to support your cycle.

We have looked at managing your pain and the various natural remedies you can use. We now move on to look at healing and supporting your immune system ... and we start with something called the Healing Crisis so that you are aware of this natural process

Understanding The 'Healing Crisis'

This is a common phenomenon and one that any natural health practitioner should prepare you for, and that is the phase of healing called the 'healing crisis'. It is something I went through myself when I was going through my own healing journey. It is totally natural and it is your body off-loading years of physical, mental and emotional ill-health that has not been addressed. Once you start a healing or detox program then your body goes into a bit of a crisis. Something very similar happens when you suddenly stop using caffeine or sugar and you can go through withdrawal.

The elimination process is often referred to as the 'healing crisis.' The word crisis sounds a bit strong as it implies an emergency, but it the best way to describe what the body is going through. Most main-stream doctors do not recognise or identify the action of a healing-crisis, but it is part of a process produced by the body to maintain survival and try to get to equilibrium.

Once the healing crisis starts, reactions may be mild or moderate. Expect ups and downs as it takes a while to start recovering your health. In a healing crisis, every body system works together to eliminate waste products and set the stage for regeneration.

Symptoms of the healing crisis may at first be identical to the disease it is meant to heal. But there is an important difference - old toxins are being eliminated. A cleansing, purifying process is underway and stored wastes are moving through the body. Sometimes pain and symptoms during the healing crisis are more intense than that of the chronic disease, but it is temporary.

An initial healing crisis usually lasts around three to five days but if the energy of the person is low, it may last a week or more. To support the detox time, your body needs fluids, and especially water to help carry off the toxins. This is a time for rest. Be kind to yourself --- mentally, emotionally, and of course physically.

This healing crisis may be noticeable if you start on a regime of treatment with any of the natural therapies like herbalism, Traditional Chinese Medicine, Naturopathy etc., and even doing an Elimination diet will cause a similar reaction.

Sometimes you may go through more than one detox stage, and with each phase symptoms will begin to improve. Go as slowly as your body can cope so your elimination is gradual and comfortable. Again, I stress the importance of drinking plenty of fluids. Support the detox process with Epsom Salts baths, skin brushing, getting fresh-air and doing some gentle exercise like walking or yoga. Just be gentle with yourself and don't be concerned about this process – it's a good sign that it is working.

Fascinating Stuff About Healing - And Do We Make Our Own Reality?

Say what ....!

I briefly want to provide you with an insight into the nature of healing and the 'reality' of the immune-system, including some scientific insights, without going all woo-woo on you! Hopefully you may find this eye-opening reading.

Before we continue, I feel it is valid to look at some of the factors within ourselves that can leave us open to becoming diseased. No blame here - just a look at how human nature can be fickle regards our health.

Through illness the body is giving us a message, telling us that something is out of balance. This is not punishment for bad behaviour, rather it is nature's way of creating equilibrium. By listening to the message, we have a chance to contribute to our own healing, and work with our body in bringing it back to a state of balance.

The word 'remission' is used to describe a period of recovery, when an illness or disease diminishes. A person is described as being 'in remission' when their symptoms decline.

There is a distinction to be made between curing and healing. To cure is to fix a particular problem and Western medicine is particularly good at doing this, by offering drugs and surgery so that disease, illness or physical problems can be repressed, eliminated or removed.

It does play a vital role in alleviating suffering, and is superb at saving lives and applying curative aid. But this only goes as far as being without symptoms in many cases. This does not always mean being without disease. Modern medicine usually means you are without symptoms, but the underlying disease can still be present.

This is where we enter the realm of healing. 'If you look no further than getting rid of what is wrong, you may never deal with what has brought your life to a standstill' says a patient in Marc Barasch's book 'The Healing Path'. To be healed means to become whole. This is not possible if we are only concerned with the individual part that needs to be cured. With endometriosis, more than just the womb and reproductive organs need to be healed.

Illness confronts us with many questions. We have choices - we can take a pill and carry on as before, or we can begin to become whole and become the person we truly wish to be.

'You need to re-assess to reclaim your health and your life'

It is only when we begin to make changes in our life, that we will be able to accomplish true and valid healing. There is no point building a solid house, if the foundations are not secure.

Your Body Is Amazing!

*Let us first look at some facts about the body to emphasise
the point that the body is indeed amazing.*

The brain itself is very, very complex, and most of its capabilities and capacities we do not understand. We only use a small portion of its potential. To duplicate the memory portion would require a computer in excess of the size of the Empire State Building.

If all our muscles pulled together in one direction, we could lift as much as 25 tons. Actually, in times of need, men and women have, without stopping to think about it, lifted weight far beyond what is usually considered possible.

Every day our blood travels 12,000 miles. Red blood cells make approximately 250,000 round trips of the body before returning to the bone marrow, where they were born, to then die. We have enough carbon for 9,000 lead pencils, and enough calcium to completely whitewash a chicken coop.

Constant Renewal

Every five days our whole intestinal lining is renewed. You make a new liver every 6 weeks. A new skin once a month. Every six months we have a new bloodstream. A complete new set of bones within 2 years. Even our brain cells are replaced. The DNA that holds memories of millions of years of evolution, even that is replaced every six weeks.

These facts left me musing on the whole concept of disease and how the body malfunctions. Why would we replace our old cells with 'newly diseased' cells? Why are we not replacing *all* our old cells with good new healthy ones?

So, it seems evident that what is happening is that our cells have memories, and we replace the new ones to be just like the old ones. Not the way that nature intended, but the way WE intended.

We start to enter the subject of our perceptions of reality. That tricky question of - do we make our own reality. We do not need to go into that topic here. That is not the aim of the advice here.

To continue........

Can you get a grasp what I am saying here about us putting back *diseased* cells in our body, when we have the chance to put *healthy* new cells into our body? Have we conditioned ourselves to respond to memories in a certain way? We can become convinced by our diseased state. As long as a person is convinced by their symptoms, they are caught up in a reality where being sick is the dominant input.

I have had feedback from a couple of women who had endometriosis with accounts of their own recovery coming about because they stopped focusing on their disease. Yes, they did take action to look after their own health, but by getting engrossed in other areas of their lives, they found that their endometriosis stopped taking centre stage and started to regress.

We do have infinite choices at every second to alter the shape of our world; our perception of our world. But through old, outdated programming we keep on creating the same old patterns in life. Habits are hard to break and our bodies are a mirror image of our thoughts.

We can heal ourselves superbly and the body does a brilliant job if it is given the chance. To repeat the quote from Deepak Chopra from his book '*Quantum Healing*':

'.......... we already know that the living body is the best pharmacy ever devised. It produces diuretics, painkillers, tranquillisers, sleeping pills, antibiotics, and indeed everything that is manufactured by the drug companies, but it makes them much, much, better. The dosage is always right and given on time; side effects are minimal or non-existent; and the directions for using the drug are included in the drug itself, as part of its built-in intelligence.'

Your Remarkable Immune System

The immune system is much more complex than most of us realise. It now appears that the immune system goes far beyond providing protection for the body from invading organisms simply through chemical processes.

I want to quote a sizeable section from a lecture given by Deepak Chopra, M.D. which is titled 'What is the True Nature of Reality? *The Basics of Quantum Healing.* This is utterly fascinating reading.

'About 20 years ago it was discovered that our thoughts and our feelings have physical substrate to them. When you think a thought, you make a molecule. To think is to practise brain chemistry. And in fact, these thoughts are translated into very precise molecules known as neuropeptides. 'Neuro' because they were first found in the brain; and 'peptides' because they are protein-like molecules. And thoughts, feelings, emotions and desires translate into the flux of neuropeptides in the brain.

You can think of these neuropeptides like little keys that fit into very precise locks called receptors on the cell walls or other neurons. So, the way this part of the brain speaks to another part of the brain is in the precise language of these neuropeptides

What was found subsequently, which was absolutely fascinating was that there were receptors to neuropeptides not only in brain cells but other parts of the body as well. So when scientists started looking for receptors to neuropeptides in cells of the immune system, for example: T cells, B cells, monocytes, and macrophages - when they started looking at them, they found that on the cell walls of all these there were receptors for the same neuropeptides which are the molecule substrate of thought.

<u>So, your immune cells are in fact constantly eavesdropping on your internal dialogue. Nothing that you say to yourself, which you are doing all the time, even in sleep, escapes the attention of the immune cells.</u> Not only that, the immune cells, it was subsequently discovered, make the same peptides that the brain makes when it thinks. Now here we come to a startling finding because if the immune cell is making the same chemicals that the brain is making when it thinks, then the immune cell is a thinking cell. It is a conscious little being.

In fact, the more you look at it, the more you find that it behaves just like a neuron. It makes the same chemical cords that the brain uses for emotion, thought, felling and desire. An immune cell has emotions. It has desires. It has intellect.

It knows how to discriminate and remember. It has to decide when it sees a carcinogen, 'Is this a carcinogen? Should I go after it? Should I leave it alone? Is this a friendly bacteria? Should I go after it or leave it alone?' It has to remember the last time it encountered something. In fact, it remembers the last time somebody else encountered the same thing.

Your immune cells can immediately recognise anything that has ever been encountered by any living species. If you are exposed to pneumococus for the first time in your life, your immune cells still remember the last time somebody somewhere in prehistoric time encountered a pneumococus and knows how to make the precise antibody to it.

It is not only a thinking cell but it remembers way back into evolutionary history of not only the human species but other species as well. So, you ask a good neurologist the difference between an immune cell and a neuron and they will say there isn't any. The immune cell is a circulatory nervous system.

Now if that wasn't enough of a startling discovery, the subsequent discoveries in science have been even more interesting, because when scientists started looking elsewhere in the body, they found the same phenomenon. When they looked at stomach cells and intestinal cells, they found the same peptides.

The stomach cells make the same chemical cords that the brain makes when it thinks. Of course, they are not verbally as elite as the brain, in that they don't think in English or Swahili, but nonetheless, they are thinking cells. When you say, 'I have a gut feeling about such and such,' you are not speaking metaphorically anymore.

You are speaking quite literally because your gut makes the same chemicals as the brain makes when it thinks. In fact, your gut feelings may be a little bit more accurate because gut cells have not yet evolved to the stage of self-doubt. (We have touched on this elsewhere with regard for the need to look after your gut health)

What science is discovering is that we have a thinking body. Every cell in our body thinks. Every cell in our body is actually a mind. Every cell has its own desires and it communicates with every other cell. The new work is not mind and body connection, we have a body-mind simultaneously everywhere.'

To finish this topic, I just want to quote one smaller section from this same lecture by Deepak Chopra, to give you another insight, or even a quick reality jolt about the nature of our being, our existence.

'............ If you could see the body as a physicist could see it, all you'd see is atoms. And if you could see the atoms as they really are, not through the artefact of sensory experience, you would see these atoms of particles that are moving at lightning speeds around huge empty spaces. These particles aren't material objects at all. They are fluctuations of energy and information in a huge

void of energy and information. If I could see your body not through this sensory artefact, I'd see a huge empty void with a few scattered dots and a few random electrical discharges here and there. 99.999999% of your body is empty space! And the .000001% of it that appears as matter is also empty space.'

Deepak Chopra goes on to explain that all this 'empty space is a fullness of non-material intelligence ...... or information that influences its own expression.' The tone of his whole lecture is to knit together ideas about the nature of the mind, the body and the nature of reality. Not an easy range of subjects individually, never mind trying to put them altogether.

Deepak mentions that we have a thinking body and that every cell thinks; this equates to what I said earlier about our bodies being a mirror image of our thoughts. What we think becomes manifest in our lives.

I feel that what Deepak Chopra reveals is extremely thought provoking with regard to how we perceive and understand the nature of our bodies and how they work. We are still only in our infancy with respect to understanding how the body really works.

Supporting Your Immune System

The immune-system is your greatest in-built asset to help you fight endometriosis and improve your overall health. It is well known that women with endometriosis tend to suffer from various other illnesses or diseases, and this is obviously a reflection of a compromised immune-system. Consequently, supporting your immune-system is a major component to recovering your health.

As we covered in the introduction, many women have endometrial tissue that strays into the abdominal cavity, but this tissue is mopped up by a healthy immune-system. But if your immune-system is not working as it should, then these stray cells may go on to develop into endometriosis. But as we do not know the true cause of this disease, we cannot totally rely on this theory, but having a strong immune is obviously going to be of benefit to sustain your overall health.

The work of your immune-system

The immune-system is designed to defend you against millions of bacteria, microbes, viruses, toxins and parasites that would normally invade your body. It works around the clock in thousands of different ways, but it does its work largely unnoticed. One thing that causes us to really notice our immune-system is when it fails for some reason.

Remedies To Support Your Immune-System

You can support your immune-system with various remedies, which can be helpful when you are under stress and trying so hard to manage disease. Many of these remedies have multiple benefits, some of which we have covered already.

Echinacea - A well-known folk remedy, Echinacea is commonly used to support the immune-system and is often the first remedy used in herbal medicine to help with colds and flu. The major benefit for echinacea is its ability to increase the number of white blood cells and is a great herb to help remove microbial infections from the body. However, echinacea should not be taken by those with auto-immune diseases as it can stimulate the immune-system and make symptoms worse.

Frankincense - This resin is gaining popularity due to its therapeutic and healing benefits. Frankincense is really helpful for calming stress and anxiety, as well as helping manage pain and inflammation. The essential oil can help calm the central nervous system and in turn help with sleep. This is a good oil to mix with Copaiba oil which will give you a great anti-inflammatory and pain-relieving blend.

Frankincense helps to support the immune-system as it has antimicrobial effects that protect from harmful bacteria and viruses. It is even reported to help fight against cancer by reducing abnormal cell growth.

The resin of frankincense is also available as a supplement called Boswellia which is helpful for endometriosis as it is shown to dramatically reduce inflammation. Additionally, Boswellia helps to boost the immune-system as well as modulate an overactive immune-system. It is also noted for helping to speed wound healing and can help with pain. It is recommended to take one capsule a day with food.

Turmeric – The spice of turmeric, as we have already covered, is often used by those with endometriosis to help with pain and inflammation and it can also support the immune-system.

Turmeric boosts the immune-system through anti-oxidant, anti-inflammatory, and anti-microbial properties. Studies have shown Turmeric to have anti-carcinogenic properties due to the active compound called Curcumin.

Healing benefits of Turmeric include boosting white blood cells, detoxifying the body and help aid restful sleep. It is best to take turmeric as a capsule which has black pepper added as this aids in absorption and taken at meal time.

Ginseng - Ginseng has the ability to increase the production of T-lymphocytes in your body. These cells are very important when it comes to your body defence mechanism. Ginseng can also help with fibromyalgia, chronic fatigue and also has anti-inflammatory benefits.

Elderberry - The berries from this herb can boost the immune-system, but caution is needed if you have an auto-immune disease, as elderberry can stimulate the immune-system and may increase symptoms.

154

Otherwise, if you have no auto-immune disease issues, then elderberry can be very supportive for your system.

Green tea - The health benefits of this tea are mentioned elsewhere and worth adding here for its immune-system benefits. Green tea can help fight diseases and infections and one of its benefits is the ability to increase the amount of interferon (immune-system proteins) produced by your liver.

Vitamin C - This vitamin is well known to help support the immune-system. It helps to support the immune-system by protecting the integrity of cells, and helps to heal wounds and sustain healthy tissues. Vitamin C acts as a strong anti-oxidant and helps to increase the production of white blood cells in the body, which are key players in your immune-system.

Zinc - Zinc is a trace element that is necessary for a healthy immune-system. A lack of zinc can make you more susceptible to disease and illness. It is responsible for a number of functions in the human body, and it helps stimulate the activity of at least 100 different enzymes. The body needs zinc to activate lymphocytes (T cells), which are needed to regulate the immune response. Foods that are high in zinc include beans, lentils, nuts, seeds and shell-fish.

Other Nutrients To Support Your Immune System

Additional dietary nutrients that are needed to support your immune-system include vitamin B12, which is needed for brain health, vitamin B complex which also helps support cognition and brain health, and finally a full spectrum of minerals.

Glutathione – your master antioxidant and immune system support

Glutathione is the body's master antioxidant, meaning it helps protect your cells from pathogens such as viruses and toxins. It also lowers the risk of developing food and chemical sensitivities, and is a powerful supporter of your immune-system. Optimal glutathione levels are also needed to assist detoxing excess estrogens and will help reduce inflammation.

Making sure your glutathione status is healthy will also support energy, brain focus and concentration. Unfortunately, environmental toxins, chronic stress, unhealthy diets, inflammation, medications, alcohol and many other factors continually deplete glutathione.

Supplements that support Glutathione

- Alpha lipoic acid
- NAC (N-acetyl-cysteine)

- SAMe (S-adenosylmethionine)
- Milk Thistle - helps reduce depletion

Glutathione can be taken as a supplement but the body does not absorb glutathione that well when using most oral supplements. The most bioavailable supplement is a liquid liposomal form of glutathione. Liposomal delivery is a more efficient way to take supplements like glutathione because it protects the therapeutic molecules from breaking down in your digestive system. Liposomal glutathione can be rather expensive, but you may feel that the broad range of benefits is worth the investment, and is one supplement I do recommend especially when you are dealing with a lot of stress putting strain on your entire system.

One of the most powerful way to increase glutathione is with coffee enemas which can increase your glutathione by 700% but I find many with endometriosis are reticent to do coffee enemas, however they are very powerful for healing and excellent for supporting the liver.

Endorphins and the immune system

Most immune cells have receptors for endorphins and need endorphins to function properly and research shows people with chronic illness have low endorphin levels. Low endorphin production can be caused by drug use, anxiety, depression, severe illness and chronic psychological stress – all of which are factors that can tip the immune system out of balance.

Low dose naltrexone, which we covered earlier, can boost your natural endorphin production which also helps to balance your immune-system.

More Ways To Support Your Immune System

Reduce stress

This is not always easy to do when you suffer from ongoing pain and distress caused by disease. Stress can really do a number on your immune-system, so you need to do all you can to manage your stress levels and the negative hormones that can be released due to stress.

Try some meditation exercises which will help to calm you down and relax your central nervous system. You will find many helpful mediation videos on YouTube. Yoga is another way to help reduce your stress levels. Additionally, try some calming teas like Chamomile or Vervain, or a few drops of CDB oil can be very helpful to help with anxiety, stress as well as pain.

Some of the essential oils that are helpful for stress and anxiety include Lavender, Chamomile, Neroil, Ylang ylang, Vetiver and Bergamot (which can also help to balance hormones). Make up a blend of oils and apply to your inner wrists and the soles of your feet.

If you find that your brain is running round in circles and you cannot switch off, then a dose of Theanine will help as it is a calming amino acid that helps to calm the brain. You can also find theanine in green tea, so another reason to be drinking this healthy tea.

Earthing

Using the simple therapy of earthing can help to balance hormones as well as support your immune-system and help to reduce pain. During recent decades, chronic illness, immune disorders, and inflammatory diseases have increased dramatically, and some researchers have cited environmental factors as the cause, such as toxic buildings, electro-magnetic pollution, constant use of tech, modern synthetic materials in the home and clothing – all of which can unbalance our system.

Using earthing sheets on your bed and using protective mats and guards when we use technology can help, as well as simply walking barefoot outside. Earthing sheets can be purchased as single or double bed size and are plugged into the power outlet of your house, without connecting to the actual power source by using a special adaptor.

Using earthing sheets are also reported to help improve sleep. It is also a good idea to get protection when using your laptop by using an EMF/radiation protection mat, and you probably know you can get covers to use with your mobile to reduce EMF risk – it's worthwhile using one to protect your health.

I personally use an EMF protection mat while using my laptop, use an earthing sheet on the bed, and I also switch off the wi-fi at bed-time to reduce radiation exposure – every little bit helps.

Sleep

Getting enough sleep is going to help support your immune-system, but I know from experience how difficult this can be when you suffer from pain and hormone disturbances. Our bodies release some important compounds while we sleep, including cytokines which help the immune-system in warding off inflammation. If you have difficulty sleeping try some of the herbs suggested in the insomnia section, especially those calming herbs that can also help with pain like Wild Lettuce and Chamomile

Supporting your immune-system is achieved by looking after your body on many fronts. Most of these ideas many seem quite obvious, but sometimes we just need a reminder. Be kind to yourself, as well as being kind to your body. Remember the earlier subject we covered about your immune-system eaves-dropping on your thoughts. Thinking positively really can help support your health.

Additional

Support

for

Your Health

> *'When you feeling like quitting, think about why you started'*

Hormone Testing

To get a clear understanding of your hormone levels it can be a good idea to have your hormones tested which will provide valuable information and take out the guess work.

Your doctor may run hormones tests which are usually blood tests. If you work with a natural therapist, they can also request hormone testing, and the type of test will depend on their training and experience. Your hormones can be evaluated with blood tests, saliva tests and dried urine test depending which hormone panel is being evaluated.

To get a complete understanding of your hormones including cortisol, DHAE and your reproductive hormones, including estrogen, testosterone, and progesterone, the Dried Urine Test for Comprehensive Hormones (DUTCH test) will give you a good overview.

The Dutch test measures your hormone metabolites from dried urine samples. Patients collect just four or five dried urine samples over a 24-hour period. Results are provided with clear charts showing reference ranges and the hormone results of each hormone being tested.

Some DUTCH tests will assess a comprehensive list of hormones, depending which laboratory is used. This usually includes:

- Cortisol
- Cortisone
- Estradiol
- Estrone
- Estriol
- Progesterone
- Testosterone
- DHEA and DHEA-S
- Melatonin

The downside regarding the DUTCH test is it tends to be rather expensive with prices ranging from $400 US to $500 for a more comprehensive test, with prices varying greatly between countries.

For those who find their doctor is unwilling to run the required tests, or you are unable to get tested through the office of a natural therapist, you have the option to order your own tests. As well as ordering your own DUTCH test, you have the option to order sex hormone blood tests which are done via a finger-prick test. You can also test your cortisol circadian rhythm with a 4-x day saliva test to check your adrenal stress response. We go into more details about cortisol testing and supporting your adrenals further on. Other tests to consider are thyroid, vitamin D and B12 and some laboratories provide these combined with female sex hormone tests. These tests tend to be more affordable than the DUTCH test and sometimes they are offered with discounts – get on their mailing list for alerts.

If you need to purchase your own tests, many laboratories will provide a doctor's report, including feedback and advice about the results of your test. I have included links at the back of the book for resources regarding hormone testing.

Progesterone Cream As Treatment

One of the ways to reduce estrogen levels and help treat endometriosis is by using natural progesterone cream. Using the cream in a sufficiently high dose can halt menstruation, similar to using synthetic hormone treatment. However, this method is less toxic than using synthetic hormones. Progesterone cream can also be used at lower doses simply to help reduce estrogen dominance.

What does progesterone do?

This advice may seem like stating the obvious for some of you, and I won't go into much detail, but briefly ....

Progesterone is secreted by the female reproductive system. Its main function is to regulate the condition of the inner lining of the uterus. Progesterone is produced by the ovaries, placenta, and adrenal glands.

A healthy woman will have the proper ratios of estrogen and progesterone each day of the month, with the ratios fluctuating depending on her age and the point in her cycle.

Progesterone also supports healthy bones and a healthy liver, heart, and brain tissue—in both women and men. In women specifically, it protects the breasts, and may reduce risk of breast cancer as well as relieve fibrocystic breast pain. It also improves, sleep, anxiety, and cholesterol.

The natural hormone progesterone is not to be confused with the synthetic hormones used in birth control pills and hormone replacement therapy. These are called progestogens, progestins or gestins. The effects of natural and synthetic hormones on the body differ enormously. The synthetics do not match the body's chemistry, so the body is not equipped to metabolise them properly.

The estrogens and progesterone in a woman's body must be in equilibrium for a woman to remain healthy. In many of us they are becoming more and more out of balance and living in a toxic environment makes matter even worse.

Treating endometriosis with progesterone

Due to the problem of estrogen dominance women are having success using natural progesterone cream to help reduce estrogen and in turn reduce the symptoms of endometriosis.

Natural progesterone cream is formulated to produce a substance that is identical to the human progesterone.

Key ways Natural Progesterone Cream will help endometriosis includes:

- Taking a high enough dose to induce a psuedo-pregnancy - this will stop the further development of endometriosis. Using Natural Progesterone Cream is a safer method to induce pseudo-pregnancy than using the synthetic Progestins which perform the same function
- Reduce further proliferation of endometriosis implants and allow any implants that are present to shrink
- Counteract estrogen dominance

Using Progesterone Cream to help endometriosis

It is advised to use the cream from day 6 of your cycle to day 26 each month, using one ounce of cream per week for three weeks, then stopping just before your expected period.

After 4 to 6 months of using the cream, women are reporting that their menstrual pains gradually subside as monthly bleeding from the endometriosis implants becomes less and healing of the inflammatory sites starts to occur.

Natural progesterone is not the same as progestin in prescription birth control pills, or the progestin used in the treatment of endometriosis. These prescription hormones are chemically modified from the natural hormones to be different in order to be patented.

Find the Correct Progesterone Cream

Many women have been led to believe Wild Yam extract cream and progesterone cream are the same thing. The fact is they are not. Many companies are marketing a cream made from wild yam extract and telling customers that their body is going to convert wild yam extract into progesterone. This is not true.

There are a number of natural progesterone creams on the market, which are being used successfully by women with endometriosis. The only successful results however are from those creams which contain a synthetic natural progesterone. This means that the progesterone being synthesised is identical to the human hormone progesterone at a molecular level. It will never be completely identical as we cannot replicate nature, but it will be as close as possible. So, this 'natural progesterone' is synthetic and is made in a laboratory.

Scientific studies have shown that for any natural progesterone cream to really be effective and increase the progesterone levels in your blood stream, there are two important factors. Firstly, a truly effective cream must contain synthetic 'natural progesterone', not wild yam extract. Secondly, to be truly effective the cream must contain a minimum of 400mg of natural progesterone per ounce.

Also be aware of any added ingredients in the cream. Some brands have been found to include various parabens, which is a group of compounds used in most toiletries, to stop the deterioration of a product. Parabens are another form of xeno-estrogen, which rather defeats the object of using the cream. You can however find Natural Progesterone Creams available that don't include parabens.

You can buy these creams OTC in some countries or purchase online at reputable websites. You apply the cream to soft tissue areas including breast, inner arms and thighs.

So do your research, and purchase the best quality Natural Progesterone Cream to help with endometriosis. These creams can be expensive and you cannot afford to be wasting your money and raising your hopes, only to find you are not getting the desired results.

Increase Your Progesterone Naturally

As well as using progesterone cream to help balance your hormones there are a number of dietary nutrients that can help boost your natural progesterone production.

Progesterone is the only hormone that is able to decrease the production of estrogen receptors in the body, diminishing the effects of estrogen and protecting our tissues.

While estrogen is stimulating in the body, natural progesterone is calming;
it's the supportive, balancing female sex hormone

How is Progesterone produced

Progesterone is produced mainly in the corpus luteum as well as the ovaries, and small amounts are also made in your adrenal glands. It is involved in the following important hormone cascade, which is critical to female hormone balance:

- Your body uses cholesterol to make pregnenolone, which is often called the 'mother of all hormones.'

- Pregnenolone is then converted into progesterone.
- Pregnenolone, is also the precursor hormone for estrogen and testosterone.
- Pregnenolone also makes other hormones including DHEA, cortisol, aldosterone, androstenedione.

The pregnenolone steal

This is a process that can happen when the body is under stress and the body 'steals' certain hormones to ensure the production of more vital hormones needed for survival like cortisol.

The pregnenolone steal is one example of an imbalanced hormonal process that can result in a range of symptoms. The pregnenolone steal can affect your body's ability to produce other hormones, including sex hormones such as progesterone, estrogen, and testosterone.

This can have downstream outcomes including:

- fatigue
- depression
- low libido
- mood swings
- irregular periods

Do some of these symptoms sound familiar? Due to the stress of managing endometriosis it is very possible you could be dealing with issues of other hormone imbalances including the pregnenolone steal. We look at ways to support the health of your adrenal glands further on, which will help to support the production of vital hormones.

Supplements to boost your progesterone production

Adding certain nutrients to your diet can help
increase your natural progesterone production.

Vitamin B6 - To increase your progesterone, a good way is to increase your vitamin B6 (pyridoxine) levels. B6 is necessary for the production of progesterone. Available as a supplement, B6 is also found in sweet potatoes, dark green leafy vegetables, sunflower seeds, tuna, salmon and poultry. As mentioned earlier, B6 also helps to reduce estrogen levels in your body.

Zinc - Zinc is essential for hormonal health and it is extremely important for the production of adequate levels of progesterone. Zinc is the mineral that prompts the pituitary gland to release follicle stimulating hormones, which in turn promote ovulation and stimulate the ovaries to produce estrogen and progesterone.

Good sources of zinc are shellfish, crab, dark chocolate, chickpeas, pumpkin, watermelon and squash seeds.

Magnesium - Magnesium plays a very important role in hormone regulation and is therefore one of the nutrients that boost progesterone levels. This is another nutrient that helps regulate the pituitary gland.

You can take dietary supplements as well as eat more foods that are good sources of magnesium such as dark leafy greens, nuts and seeds especially squash and pumpkin, mackerel, whole grains like brown rice, dark chocolate.

Vitamin C - Research has shown that women who take vitamin C have significantly increased levels of progesterone, and in research it was found that women who took 750mg of vitamin C per day had an increase of progesterone by **77** percent.

Chasteberry (Vitex) - A herb that is good for balancing hormone levels in the body is chasteberry, also known as vitex. It can stimulate progesterone production and reduce levels of estrogen, as well as amounts of prolactin, which is another hormone that can lead to low progesterone in the body.

Vitamin E - Vitamin E can help to boost progesterone levels which was reported in a study published in the Journal of Ovarian Research. Researchers found that when patients were given vitamin E, almost three-quarters of them had a significant increase in progesterone levels.

Castor Oil Packs

Castor oil packs have become very popular and have some great benefits to help the symptoms of endometriosis. They are really helpful for calming pain and inflammation when you have a flare and are very good for detoxing the liver and help shift excess estrogen. They are also able to calm the central nervous system and can be very soothing to help aid with sleep. They are also thought to be able to break down scar tissue.

Castor oil has been used therapeutically for hundreds of years, both internally and externally and have been used for numerous aliments. It has been used to treat everything from colitis and peptic ulcers to arthritis and female problems from back pain to fibroids, and PMS.

The castor oil pack is a simple procedure and to sum up their health benefits:

- Can help to reduce the bloat of endo belly
- Helps break down scar tissue
- Eases cramping when used on the abdomen
- Calms central nervous system
- Increases lymphatic flow
- Reduces inflammation, pain and swelling
- Support liver detox when placed over the liver
- Strengthens the immune system
- Supports digestion

To do a castor oil pack you require:

- 1 cotton or wool flannel cloth, about 12 inches square (a piece of old sheet is fine but make sure there are no synthetics in the fabric)
- 2 plastic sheets - one to protect the bed, one smaller to wrap around the area being treated - for endometriosis, the pack will be applied to the abdomen
- hot water bottle
- Approx. 100ml of castor oil
- bath towels
- safety pins
- hot water

Method:

- heat the castor oil in a saucepan, hot enough to put straight onto the skin without scalding. Immerse the cloth in the oil and stir round with tongs, ensuring that it gets thoroughly saturated
- meanwhile cover the bed with a plastic sheet and a large towel to protect the sheets
- lift out the saturated cloth and place it over the area to be treated. For endometriosis, the cloth needs to be placed over the central abdomen area
- now wrap the area securely in the plastic, then a towel, and secure with safety pins
- lie down carefully and lay a hot water bottle on the area being treated
- leave on overnight, or at least for 2 hours
- in the morning, strip off the pack and store in a plastic bag so that it can be reused
- after taking off the pack, you can wash the area with water and a little baking soda. This is to stop any rash from developing. Washing off the oil is not always necessary - for example, if you have just done a pack before going to bed and don't want to wear the pack overnight - just wipe off the excess with tissues and leave the rest of the oil to soak in over-night - you will get

some added benefits from the oil over night. You may get a slightly oily nightdress but it easily washes out.

Tip: I have found it easy to reuse the castor oil cloth many times - just pop it in a 'zippy' fastening poly-bag when you have finished, and it's ready to use again another time. The heat from your body combined with the heat from a hot water bottle will warm the cloth. If the cloth does not seem oily enough you can just rub some oil straight onto your skin before applying the castor oil cloth.

Try to aim for 2 to 3 sessions of treatment on consecutive nights and then rest for a few nights.

Ensure your castor oil is hexane free. (Hexane free castor oil is a natural castor oil that does not use any harmful chemicals during the extraction process and is free of all synthetic chemicals).

* It is advised not to do a castor oil pack when you are menstruating, or if you are pregnant.

Remove Toxins To Aid Your Health

It is *highly* recommended that you start to remove toxins from your system, which will help improve your overall health and also help improve your symptoms. When you change to using more natural products you will reduce your toxic load and reduce the amount of xeno-estrogens and chemicals from entering your system. Women have reported to me that they are quite surprised how much difference it has made to their health when they started using natural products.

Xeno-estrogens

Xeno-estrogens can mimic estrogen in your body, which as we known can worsen symptoms of endometriosis. These synthetic compounds can be found in your food, in packaging, toiletries, household cleaners, plastics and in pesticides.

There is increasing evidence and research which report how these chemicals can really mess with your hormones and your endocrine system. It can sometimes seem impossible to avoid all these toxins in the environment.

Fortunately, there are now many companies that product safer cleaning products as well as safer cosmetics and toiletries.

Period products

Another product you are advised to change is your period products and use organic versions instead of the usual commercial products. Period products also contain many chemicals and then you put them next to your skin! Some products have been found to contain dioxins, which as we have covered, have a very detrimental effect on health, especially for endometriosis.

Cookware

One area regarding toxins that can be overlooked is modern cookware, like Teflon and non-stick pans which can leach chemicals into your food every time you cook. Safer options include stainless steel or cast-iron. We covered this topic earlier in 'Utensils for cooking' if you need a reminder.

Toxic Ingredients In Toiletries

Our skin is the largest organ and absorbs everything

To give you an idea just how toxic toiletries are, this list should convince you to change over to natural alternatives. Some of these chemicals arrive at the production facility with the 'skull & cross-bones' sticker – ***this tells you just how lethal they are!***

Sodium Lauryl Sulphate (SLS) - Found in shampoos, hair conditioners, toothpastes, body washes, strong detergent which can cause eye irritation, permanent damage to the eyes, especially in children, skin rashes, hair loss, flaking skin and mouth ulceration.

When combined with other ingredients, can form nitrosamines, which are carcinogenic. Easily penetrates the skin and can lodge itself in the heart, lungs, liver and brain. SLS can damage the immune system; causing separation of skin layers and inflammation of skin.

Fluoride - linked to cancer deaths and can badly affect the thyroid.

Propylene Glycol - used in anti-freeze, paint, floor wax - used in many personal care products.

Isopropyl - This is a poisonous solvent and denaturant (alters the structure of other chemicals) and can be found in toiletries. Isopropyl dries hair and skin, creates cracks and fissures in the skin, which encourages bacterial growth and can cause headaches, flushing, nausea, vomiting and depression.

Petrolatum & Mineral Oil - This is used industrially as a petroleum-based grease component and is also known as liquid Vaseline. This substance strips the natural oils from the skin and forms an oily film over the skin, which prohibits the release of toxins. It can also cause photosensitivity, chapping, dryness and premature ageing.

Parabens - *parabens have estrogenic effects on the body*, and parabens are found in nearly all toiletry products. As a result, using commercial, chemical-based toiletries will increase the levels of estrogen in the body and in turn may add to the further development of endometriosis.

Safe Toiletry Options

Women have provided me with feed-back which validates the fact that when they stop using chemical-based toiletries their health improves, and their symptoms of endometriosis start to improve as well. By cutting out these toxic toiletries and using natural, safer alternatives they are able to eliminate these toxins and xeno-estrogens from their bodies.

To avoid most of the toxic chemicals of commercial toiletries, it is now possible to purchase safe, chemical free products. Shopping online is a good starting point which allows you to see if there are any feedback reviews about particular products.

The range of quality natural toiletries is increasing all the time with many promoting their products being chemical free as well as organic. Do check all the ingredients before you purchase, as some companies are advertising their products as being safe and free of chemicals, while they may actually contain unwanted chemicals.

If you are unsure about a particular ingredient then look it up online, because some ingredients may sound nasty using their technical name, whereas they are actually just natural ingredients with a nasty sounding name.

You also have the option to produce some of your own simple toiletries, which can easily be done in your own kitchen. Most of these preparations use common ingredients, some of which may already be in your kitchen cupboards. Just look online and you will find plenty of recipes for making your own beauty care products.

Moisturisers

It starts with water …..

Water is the secret ingredient for dewy-fresh skin. Water moves through the body to the surface in a process called 'trans-epidermal water loss' leaving skin pleasingly plump and firm. If your system is deficient in water, the skin's upper layers become dry and brittle.

Drinking at least six glasses of water daily and eating fluid-rich fruits and vegetables helps to normalise dry or oily skin, and is essential for preventing your body from robbing its necessary moisture at the expense of your skin.

A wide variety of commercial moisturisers are available on the market that range from the inexpensive to ridiculously expensive. However, most of these products contain added ingredients to help maintain shelf life, stop oxidization, and many products include those toxic parabens.

Essential Oils for beauty

Essential oils are a great option for making a natural moisturizer or body oil. Most commercial moisturisers soothe and sit on the surface of the skin, but essential oils with their fine molecular structure work their way through from the surface to the inner dermis. This has the benefit of allowing the healing properties of essential oils to penetrate into the skin as well as the blood stream.

My own oil of choice to use as a carrier oil for essential oils, is Almond oil, as it does not feel too heavy and is reasonably priced. A rule of thumb for adding essential oils to a carrier oil is - 30ml of base oil with 6 to 8 drops of essential oil. You can use more than one type of essential oil per mix, but divide the number of drops so that the combined number still totals 6 to 8 drops to 30ml of base oil - you will not gain anything by making the mixture stronger.

Different Oils for Skin Care

- Fragile capillaries: Lemon, Camomile, Cypress, Lavender
- Dermatitis: Sage, Camomile, Hyssop, Geranium
- Eczema, dry: Juniper, Lavender, Geranium
- Eczema, weeping: Juniper, Camomile, Bergamot
- Mature skin: Rose, Lavender, Clary-sage, Frankincense
- Inflamed: Clary-sage, Camomile, Lavender, Geranium
- Dry: Camomile, Lavender, Geranium, Neroli, Sandalwood
- Oily: Bergamot, Lemon, Geranium, Cypress, Cedarwood
- Rejuvenating: Lavender, Melissa, Frankincense, Jasmine

You can use a mixture of oils to suit your skin type or address any skin problems. If you use an essential oil blend on your skin every night you will soon see improvements in the health of your skin.

Natural Hair Colour

*A way to perk up hair (and perk up yourself) is by
changing the colour of your hair*

However, as well as the toxic effects caused by the chemicals in modern chemical hair colours, they also do a lot of damage to the structure of the hair. These chemicals will permeate through your pores and will then circulate in your system upsetting your natural hormone balance as well as causing additional damage.

Natural hair products

Commercial <u>natural</u> dyes have become more popular, offering a wide range of colours, often using herbs and natural oils in their products. Because natural hair dyes gradually fade, you do not have to worry about touching up the roots. Be sure to read the list of ingredients carefully, since some companies 'cheat' by combining plant dyes with strong chemical dyes.

Henna hair dye

Henna hair dye is another option for colouring your hair without chemicals, and comes in a variety of different shades. Henna has been used throughout India, Egypt and the Middle East for a few thousand years to give hair a red highlight and condition it.

It can take many hours for henna to take, but it is much safer than using chemicals. It coats dry hair with a vegetable protein that makes it shiny with extra body, and it can actually help with oily hair. Some people are sensitive to henna, so do a patch test on your inner arm before trying this herb on your hair.

Natural Deodorant

If you shop around you can buy sulphate and paraben free deodorants or you can try one of the natural crystal deodorant stones. Crystal deodorant is a type of alternative deodorant made of natural mineral salt called potassium alum. Crystal deodorant is available as a stone, roll-on, or spray. Sometimes you can find it as a gel or powder. They are readily available online or from health shops.

Perfume Options

Finding a quality perfume these days often means you have to pay a lot of money, and what you are really paying for is the cost of the extravagant marketing and glitzy packaging of the products you buy.

You always have the option of using essential oils – just think of Jasmin, Sandalwood, Vetiver and Ylang Ylang all of which have delicious scents and you get health benefits from the oil into the bargain.

Essential oils are also a simple and safe way to add some lovely scents to your home by adding a few drops to water in an essential oil burner. Burning lavender oil is very beneficial as it is able to reduce air-borne germs as well as being very calming.

Nutrients needed to support hair growth

I thought I would pop this snippet of advice in here as I know many of you suffer from hair problems and falling hair due to endometriosis.

The health of your hair can be one of the first things that suffers when you are dealing with ill-health. We have looked at the problem of low iron and how it can be very detrimental to your overall health when it is low, and can include the health of your hair. Also, having low thyroid levels will cause serious hair-loss, including your eye-brows as well as the hair on your head. This is why you need to get ALL your hormones checked, and to not think all your symptoms are caused by endometriosis.

Nutrients needed to support healthy hair growth:

Biotin - commonly used as a hair growth supplement

Zinc - zinc plays an important role in hair tissue growth and repair

Vitamin A - needed for growth

Vitamin D - thought to play a role in hair production

Iron - this is definitely needed for hair growth and having endometriosis can cause heavy periods which could lead to low iron levels

Horsetail - a great source of organic silicon. This mineral helps give elasticity, firmness and resistance to hair.

Collagen - helps to support healthy hair and aids in soft supple skin

Hair growth spray

*Here is a recipe for a spray to help
promote hair growth and increase strength*

Make a mixture rosemary and cedar-wood essential oils mixed with a few drops of witch hazel and water. Put mixture in a spray bottle and spray on daily, massaging gentle into the scalp.

Two other natural remedies used to support healthy hair that get rave reviews include Brahmi oil, an Ayurveda remedy to promote hair growth, which is applied to the scalp. The other remedy is Jamaican black castor oil, which is also used by massaging onto the scalp and the hair. You will find lots of videos on YouTube about using these remedies.

Safe Ways To Clean Your Home

The following advice gives you some tips and ideas to keep your home clean without using a multitude of different chemical-based products.

People often invest in separate products for individual cleaning jobs: furniture polish, bathroom floor cleaner, kitchen surface cleaner, oven cleaner, bleach for general purpose around the house, 2-3 laundry detergents for cleaning clothes, glass cleaner, drain cleaner - the list goes on.

If you look in the average cleaning cupboard of many homes, you will find a huge array of different bottles, cans and containers; some of which may have only been used once. Some of them will be past their 'use by date', and you have to throw it away - more toxic garbage thrown into the environment - and you have wasted your money.

You may also notice that many products advise to keep away from children or your pets, must be used in a well-ventilated room, and many will have severe warning logos stamped on the container, which means they are either highly toxic or flammable and down-right dangerous.

All of these products are costly, dangerous to your home, family and the environment. You can keep your home clean, germ free and smelling sweet by using only 2-3 home-made organic products, and you will save money.

Let's start with the kitchen

Rather than use a different cleaning product for the stove, kitchen sink, cabinets, floor and refrigerator, work tops and so on, there are only 4 ingredients that you need, and you can purchase them in any grocery store. They are: **white vinegar, baking soda, lemon juice and salt.**

Also take note - all of those ingredients you can put into your mouth quite safely without fear of poisoning.

- Kitchen Floors - In a bucket mix 1/2 cup white vinegar with 1-gallon hot water. This is safe for hardwood, linoleum, tile, and any washable surface.
- Oven Cleaner - Mix 1 tablespoon of baking soda, 1 tablespoon salt, and add 1/2 cup hot water. Make a gritty paste, apply to the oven, heat slightly, cool and then wipe away with a damp rag.
- Refrigerator Seals - The plastic seals of refrigerators can be wiped free of debris with a rag dabbed in white vinegar.
- Kitchen Cabinets - 1/4 cup of lemon juice mixed with 1 quart of hot water. Lemon juice helps to remove grease from wood and metal.

The bathroom

The same cleaning products used in the kitchen are suitable for the bathroom; white vinegar, baking soda, and lemon juice.

- To clean the toilet, sprinkle in baking soda and scrub with a toilet brush
- Bathroom Glass Cleaner-1-2 tablespoons of white vinegar mixed with 1 quart of water in a spray bottle. To remove oily or greasy fingerprints from the mirror, dab on a little rubbing alcohol and wipe with a linen rag.
- Bathroom Floors-The same as kitchen floors: 1/2 cup of vinegar with 1-gallon hot water. This is safe for hardwood, linoleum, tile, and any washable surface.

Other cleaning areas

To polish wood furniture and wood floors, and to have a wonderful citrus scent, use citrus oil. You can purchase citrus oil from many home-improvement stores

- Polishing Wood Furniture - pour a small amount of citrus oil (undiluted) onto a lint-free rag, and polish to perfection.
- Another Furniture Polish - mix equal parts olive oil and lemon juice for a natural furniture polish. Just apply with a soft cloth and buff to a shine.

A few more household tips to minimise your need for toxic chemical-based preparations:

- Throw away your air freshener and try herbal bouquets, pure vanilla on a cotton ball, essential oils used with a special burner, or perhaps try opening the windows - even if it is a bit chilly.
- Clean window/mirrors/glass by adding a little vinegar and a little liquid soap to a spray bottle of water. Shake mixture a little and spray on surface that needs cleaning, and clean/polish with soft cloths.
- Drains - pour a cup of baking soap and a cup of vinegar down the drain followed by a quart of boiling water, to deodorise and keep flowing freely.

These are just a few of the ways you can use simple safe ingredients to keep your home clean. How do you think our Grandmothers managed ....? Easy, by using the methods above.

Chuck out all those bottles of toxic cleaners. Your basic cleaning shopping list will be as follows: Vinegar, Baking Soda, Lemon Juice, Salt

Problems With Period Products

Modern menstrual products can cause problems for women's health but can be even worse when suffering endometriosis.

Conventional menstrual products pose a problem for women's health because they are full of harmful chemicals. Whether using tampons or pads, many of the products on the shelves contain ingredients like bleach, dioxins, furans and even pesticide residues. You are then wearing these products close to your skin on the most delicate part of your body.

These chemicals found in feminine hygiene products have been linked to cancer, reproductive issues and hormone disruption. There are other chemicals that have been found in certain products and I shall just mention the worst ones here – and suffice to say, these products are very toxic.

Some of the chemicals in period products include:
- Glyphosate (Round-up): cancer-causing
- Chloroform: disease-causing, hormone-disrupting, a neurotoxin
- Styrene: cancer-causing
- Chloromethane: hormone-disrupting
- Chloroethane: cancer-causing
- Acetone: irritates the skin

These harmful chemicals can really disrupt your hormones and nervous system. Introducing these chemicals into your system when suffering endometriosis is like throwing fuel onto the fire. Your hormones are already thrown out of whack and adding these chemicals and toxins into your system will only make matters worse.

Problem with tampons

Tampon fibres are often bleached, so they can alter the natural pH of your vagina. They also affect the tissue elasticity of your vagina, so stopping the use of tampons can help to keep your skin healthy and elastic. Additionally, tampons can be very irritating and drying, which can become very uncomfortable. Because they can contribute to yeast growth, tampons can make cases of Candida worse.

What are your alternatives

Thankfully, there are many alternative options to conventional menstrual products.

The synthetic materials used to make these products, like plastics and rayon, are often bleached, and contain residue of pesticides and herbicides. Additional toxins are used in production like chlorine, deodorants, fragrances, and glues. These chemicals can contribute to cancer and hormone imbalances.

It is also worth noting that many modern period products are not biodegradable and can take a staggering 250 to 500 years to biodegrade. This is another reason to be looking for safe and natural alternatives.

Safe Period Products

Organic Cotton Tampons

Organic tampons look and act the same as non-organic ones, but they don't contain harmful chemicals. They are unbleached and made using organic cotton without cancer-causing additives like plastics, glues, pesticides, fragrances, or chlorine.

Organic Cotton Pads or Cloth Pads

Organic cotton pads are a popular option with the endometriosis community. Organic pads are made with organic cotton without the use of any bleaching agents. They offer the same protection as a regular pad, but without the toxins.

Reusable pads

Many companies have sprung up that make reusable pads which are made from cotton. Most women buy a variety of pads of different thicknesses and absorption. You then rinse them through when you want to change. The idea of using these products may seem strange at first but this was the way woman used to protect themselves in the past.

The Menstrual Cup

The menstrual cup is another option which is a silicone cup, inserted in the vagina, and sits just below the cervix. They come in different sizes to use for different flow rates. Similar to using tampons, the menstrual cup catches blood to stop it from leaving your body. The cup is more efficient than tampons as it does not allow blood leakage.

For the average period flow a cup can stay in place between half to a whole day without needing emptying. Once you get used to using the cup and you know your flow rate you will have a better idea of how often to empty the cup.

To sum up

Changing to more natural menstrual products is going to reduce your exposure to toxins and this will decrease any damage they may have caused to your body, as well as the upset they can cause to your hormone system. You will definitely see an improvement in your symptoms and many women have provided feedback to validate the benefits of going natural.

Benefits Of Exercise

A brief word about exercise which I know from experience can be very difficult when you have endometriosis. Whenever I had some energy, I would go for a gentle walk to get the benefits of fresh-air and sunshine. Later when my health improved, I was able to go back to horse riding which helped me greatly both physically and mentally.

If you feel up to it then try some gentle yoga exercises, do some stretching or go for a walk and get the benefits of being in nature. Getting outside is good for our mental health and helps to reduce depression. Exercise will also help to improve your circulation and can actually help to reduce your fatigue.

If you want a few ideas to get you started with some simple yoga there are tutorials on YouTube, and there are even specific videos for chair-yoga which you could try on the days when you don't feel up to doing too much physically.

Can exercise improve your symptoms?

There are good reasons why exercise will help your symptoms

- Exercise releases endorphins which are the feel-good hormones which act like natural pain relievers to lower your pain. It only takes 10 minutes of moderate exercise to release these hormones.
- Exercise improves your circulation which will help to improve blood flow to your organs. In turn this will increase your oxygen flow.

- Exercise can help to lower the amount of estrogen in your body, so exercise can help to improve your symptoms.
- Doing fifteen minutes of exercise a day can help to boost your mitochondria function which helps with energy production.
- Movement and gentle exercise improve your immune-system
- An anti-inflammatory effect takes place for a while after exercising.

Benefits Of Yoga For Endometriosis

Yoga is typically known to help with a number of conditions and usually is suggested for people who are seeking a way to de-stress and relax the mind. Yoga focuses on breathing and slow movements or poses. These poses focus on building core muscle strength and also to gain balance and re-alignment within the body.

Women with endometriosis are often easily stressed and struggle with extreme emotions. The level of pain experienced is often closely related to the associated stress levels they are currently experiencing.

Stress causes muscle tension and emotions to flare which in turn makes the pain so much worse than it needs to be. Exercise and allowing oneself to de-stress are vital to the healing of endometriosis and yoga offers one the perfect balance of both.

Yoga allows one to slow down and focus

When one's mind is travelling at a million miles an hour is it hard to really relax and even to enjoy life. Yoga helps to slow down the mind and to regain the focus on the specific task at hand, without the unnecessary stress of thinking of the future or the past.

Taking in what is happening in this moment, during a specific time is the best way to deal with specific situations. Stress is often associated with thinking and focussing on the negative too much and not being in the moment right now.

Yoga has an associated positive feeling

The poses in Yoga are focused and specific to aid in gaining balance and a sense of calm. Many of the poses will have an associated positive feeling, such as a feeling of self, power and balance and control. These are great emotions to carry with you throughout the day.

Build inner core strength

Yoga has a great way of building muscles within the body, without needing to push oneself too much. The poses use your own body weight and one can take the pose to whichever level you are able, without needing to follow repetitive, often boring methods to gain a result.

Learn to breathe properly

You would be amazed at how poorly you breathe! Breathing is crucial to getting all the necessary nutrients to get to where they need to go. When we get stressed or are rushing, check your breathing. It is likely to be shallow and short. Yoga teaches us how to breathe properly and to take time to do breathing exercises when we get stressed.

Yoga is one of the few exercises you can do at home or out in the fresh air in your garden. Once you learn the poses, they are easy to combine to create your own special morning and afternoon routine.

You will find numerous videos on YouTube with yoga instructions that are specific to help endometriosis, with many gentle routines suitable for beginners.

Pilates For Exercise

Pilates is another gentle form of exercise that is suitable for those with endometriosis.

Pilates is a form of exercise that focuses on balance, posture, strength and flexibility. A Pilates routine generally includes exercises that promote core strength and stability, muscle control and endurance, including exercises that stress proper posture and movement patterns and balanced flexibility and strength.

Pilates places a lot of focus on strengthening the core muscles. Our core muscles are the ones that stabilise our pelvis and spine in order to maintain optimum alignment. There are some similarities between Yoga and Pilates. Both systems focus on working the mind and body, with an emphasis on relaxation and breathing patterns. However, Pilates is more of a physical therapy program, whereas Yoga centres on spiritual well-being.

There is no need for any special equipment, you just need a basic floor mat similar to the mats used for yoga.

What are the benefits of Pilates?

By practicing Pilates regularly, you can achieve a number of health benefits, including:

- Improved core strength and stability
- Improved posture and balance
- Improved flexibility
- Prevention and treatment of back pain
- Pilates can focus the mind and help to reduce stress

As well as videos for yoga, YouTube also has many instructional videos for Pilates, with many aimed at beginners. You will also find a number instructional DVD's and books available giving instructions to help you do Pilates at your own pace at home.

Pain stopping you exercise?

For those who find exercise virtually impossible due to pain, this is often caused by adhesions and scar tissue in the abdominal cavity, which I know is a problem for many. To help break-down scar tissue and adhesions it can be helpful to use serrapeptase for a few months which can reduce scar tissue as well as help reduce inflammation (refer back to the topic of serrapeptase for more advice on using this supplement). Another nutrient to include is MSM, which is found naturally in the body, as it helps to keep tissue soft which can help reduce scar tissue, and can also assist with reducing inflammation.

Additionally, working with an experienced pelvic physical therapist may help to reduce scar tissue and adhesions and can also help release tight pelvic muscles. After a few treatments you will hopefully start to feel more flexibility and ease of movement. In the meantime, try to maintain some type of gentle movement, even if this means just walking round the house to help keep things moving rather than becoming totally sedentary.

ADVICE FROM AN ENDO WARRIOR

The following advice was sent to the website at Endo Resolved by Judith in Australia, to give other women some support and positive guidance - which includes 7 key suggestions to help cope with endometriosis on a day-to-day basis.

'After reading many of your own stories, mine is pretty similar. I was first diagnosed in 2015 after reading a story about endometriosis in our local newspaper. All the previous years had been a mass of unrelated pain, misdiagnosis and so called "IBS" which was not the case. A huge jigsaw puzzle finally fitting together..! Looking back over these past 13 years, heaps of surgery and treatment, there are a few things (7)! I have learned that I would like to pass on to you all. Take the advice or not - it's up to you...!

1. If you are not comfortable with your doctor, get a referral to another, before you commit to surgery or treatment.

2. Find out as much as you can about the treatments the doctors want to give you. If you are not comfortable with the treatment and its side effects, tell the doctor and ask for alternatives, only then can you make an informed decision. Don't be pressured into a decision on the spot.

3. Never be afraid to ask for help. There are support groups around the world who are there to help you. You are never alone and sometimes just talking to someone on the phone from the support group can be a great source of support and understanding for you or your family.

4. Always explore alternative therapies. These may include diet, natural therapies - including acupuncture, Chinese medicine, remedial massage, reflexology etc. Whilst some of you may or may not benefit from these types of alternate therapies, it is always worth a try! Never be afraid to change your diet and explore opportunities through natural medicines/therapies.

5. Never lose your sense of humor! Whilst endo may try to take up much of our time and energy and shorten our fuses a little too much, never forget to laugh. We all have our endo moments! That's what I call them... - We can look back at those kind of days- shake our heads and think "What in the hell was I thinking??? - or not thinking?" and take a laugh at ourselves. Or, rent or go and see a funny movie and laugh a bit. It's good therapy....

6. Don't let endo consume you... There are lots more things in life than just endo. Breathing, eating, sleeping, talking, involvement with family and friends are all other things that we can do in a day. Try not to focus on the bad things, I know that's difficult if you are in pain, but try to keep busy with things that you enjoy.

7. Keep an open mind and a positive outlook. Specific treatments both mainstream medical, drug, alternate therapies etc, may not work for everyone, but keep an open mind when considering all your options. Just because it hasn't worked for one person, doesn't mean it won't for you. Give every decision you make a good run - so that you won't look back and wish you had done things differently. Try the best you can to stay positive.

Looking back, knowing what I have learned over the years, there are probably many things I may have done differently - 20/20 vision in hindsight isn't really helpful at this point. Not all treatments work for all women. I know some of these seem pretty corny lines, but all have helped me get through my endo journey so far in one piece. Hope you find something that helps you too!'

Solutions

&

Tips

for Other

Problems

'Your body will be around a lot longer than that expensive handbag. Invest in yourself.'

Anonymous

Tips For Coming Off The Birth Control Pill

Coming off the Birth Control Pill (BCP) can be a good move to get your own hormones back on track. My own encounter with the BCP lasted about one year and other people were noticing radical changes in my mental health, but I did not notice it myself. That's probably because the change crept up on me so I did not really equate it to being on the pill. But when I stopped the pill it was like a light coming on and the heavy depressed emotional state I was in suddenly lifted.

While the BCP can help suppress some of your symptoms of endometriosis, your hormones are striving to sustain their normal balance. Taking drugs then throws a curve-ball and upsets your body, this then causes side-effects as your body becomes out of balance.

You may be suffering side effects and not really putting two and two together, possibly thinking that what you are suffering are symptoms of endometriosis. Some of the side effects may include nausea, weight gain, visual changes, decreased libido, headaches, breast tenderness and bloating – as you can see, there are comparisons to endometriosis symptoms.

You may not suffer any of these side effects, and your decision may be based on going natural and reducing your use of any drugs. Fortunately, you can stop the BCP at any time and there is no need to wean off like you would with other drugs.

However, it is a good idea to prepare for three months to support your body and ensure your body has all the nutrients it needs, as the pill can deplete your system.

You may be concerned that your endometriosis pain will come back after stopping the pill but if you support your body through detox, and adjust your nutrition to make sure you are not eating foods that can trigger pain (prostaglandins) then this will help to mitigate the changes in your body.

Birth control pill and your thyroid

Nearly 1 in 3 people have thyroid disease, the majority of whom are women

One really good reason for stopping the birth control pill is because it messes with your thyroid function. Birth control pills deplete vital nutrients your thyroid requires and can interfere with thyroid hormones on many levels.

To produce thyroid hormones your body requires selenium and zinc to convert it to the active hormone of T3. Zinc is also required for getting your thyroid hormone and cell receptors working together, and B vitamins also play an important role in thyroid function. All these nutrients are important for thyroid health and can be depleted by taking the birth control pill.

The pill also elevates Thyroid Binding Globulin (TBG) and it binds your thyroid hormones making less hormones available for your body to use. The pill also causes your body to bind up any thyroid hormone your body actually manages to make. All together the BCP is bad news for your thyroid and can lead to hypothyroidism, causing a huge list of debilitating symptoms which is a topic we will cover further on.

Here are a few tips for easing the transition

Coming off the BCP can cause a detox as your body clears itself of unwanted toxins and you need to support your body to aid in the detox process.

Support your nutrients

Certain B vitamins can become depleted by oral contraceptives, especially B2, B6, B9 and B12. A good B complex supplement will help and you need to take sublingual B12 as this vitamin is difficult to absorb via the gut. Vitamin C is another nutrient that can become depleted, and vitamin C supports your immune system and aids in the production of progesterone. Eat healthy fats as they help build healthy hormones and make sure you stay hydrated as this helps with detoxing your system.

Trace minerals

The BCP can deplete certain minerals especially selenium, magnesium and zinc. Many women are deficient in magnesium so supplementing will support your system and you can increase your intake of dark leafy greens, nuts and seeds. Selenium can also be supplemented or you can eat a few Brazil nuts which are high in selenium.

Gut microbiome

The birth control can also mess up your gut microbiome, so you need to support your gut with prebiotics and probiotics and gut healing support like colostrum and Aloe vera juice. Chicory root powder is a good prebiotic and I add it to my evening herbal tea, as prebiotics seem to be calming to the system and can aid in sleep.

Support your liver

As we have covered already, your liver is a vital organ to help off-load toxins, and coming off the pill will be another reason to support your liver. Refer back to the Liver detox section for advice on supporting your liver and add in liver supporting foods into your diet. Other ways to support the detox process is with Epsom salts baths, clean diet and castor oil packs. This is a good time to ensure you are taking

Milk Thistle and NAC to support your liver, because your liver has been working hard to process these artificial hormones.

Tracking your cycle

Once you are off the BCP it will be a good idea to start tracking your cycle and the best way to do this is with one of the apps to use on your phone. You need to start tracking your cycle from the first day of bleeding which is your first day of your cycle. You have probably been on the pill continuously for endometriosis, and will probably start bleeding soon after stopping the pill so this will be your 'day one' on your cycle.

For most women it usually takes around three months for their hormones to balance out. You need to try and keep stress levels down, because increased stress often leads to increased cortisol, and this can lead to a reduction in progesterone. Doing some light yoga exercise daily will help with stress levels and you can massage your body with some calming aromatherapy oils to help lower your stress.

To recap – nourish your body -- support your liver and detox pathways -- calm your stress reactions -- track you cycle

Keeping A Diary – Monitor Your Symptoms

I personally found the process of keeping a diary which recorded my symptoms a very useful tool. I then went on to improve my record keeping and I started to keep a visual journal by plotting symptoms on graph paper.

I found this method much more flexible rather than using one of the apps available for tracking the menstrual cycle. I wanted to track specific symptoms as well as add notes about diet, supplements taken and when I had taken any homeopathic remedies.

The reviews for these apps are very mixed and only one app I found had consistently good reviews. However, the symptoms you could track were obviously limited to the design of the app. So, designing your own method to tracking symptoms allows you to monitor what is specific to you, especially if you are starting to use natural treatments.

Charting on graph paper, recording one month per sheet, gave me a very quick 'view at a glance' of how my health was progressing. I also found that over time I was able to layout these charts on the floor and I instantly got a very quick understanding of what was happening to my symptoms and changes taking place. I used different colour felt pens for each symptom, and then wrote up any special events at the bottom of each day's entry.

I was able to be quite specific with how I rated my symptoms. For example, if I had a lot of pain, I would fill in the block completely, but if I only had medium pain, I would fill in only half the block. I used the same process for sleep (half a block for bad night - full block for full night's sleep), and for other symptoms I did the same.

The main symptoms I charted included:

- days I had periods and noted levels of blood loss
- bowel movements – because this was one symptom that really caused me issues
- pain symptoms – and noting how bad they were and at what time of day
- sleep pattern – insomnia was another bad symptom for me for a while
- energy levels – plotting whether my energy was low, medium or good
- changes in dietary intake
- notes of any new supplements taken/changes
- I also add notes of any special occasions, days I took any homeopathic remedies etc.

Maybe you prefer to use an app to track your symptoms but being a visual/creative person, I preferred the immediate method of using the old-fashioned 'pen & paper' method. You could also use a spread-sheet to design your own symptoms tracker.

Each completed sheet allowed me enough space to chart my symptoms and special notes. I could then easily view how things were developing and how life events were affecting my health. I could keep an accurate record of my menstrual cycle - I even put in the notes, the time of day that my period started. If I had a bad bout of Irritable Bowel, I would note down what I had eaten to give me a guide of what had possibly triggered it.

These visual notes can be taken to your doctor, gynaecologist or any natural health practitioner you are working with. It is a quick, simple and concise record of all your health symptoms and is a valuable tool for them as well as yourself.

I highly recommend you start to chart your health now; it may give you more clues than you realise. I kept mine pinned to a notice-board above the dresser in the bedroom, with a pot of colour pens. Using colour pens, and colouring in the blocks is quick and easy to do, and is much easier to 'read' than written notes.

Tracking my symptoms was so important to my whole healing journey and helped me keep a handle on what was helping and what was causing problems.

Help For Nausea

Nausea is a very common symptom with endometriosis, suffered by many and seems to have a number of causes. It is obvious that sometimes nausea stems from an upset in the gut and your gut can be very sensitive. We all know that sick feeling that comes with anxiety or fear.

Nausea can be really bad with endometriosis causing vomiting on a regular basis while for others it is only really acute just before and during menstruation. It is interesting to note that your body is flooded with negative prostaglandins just before menstruation and this too can cause nausea.

Neurotransmitters and pain

Reducing pain can help to reduce nausea, which may sound obvious. Here are a few tips to help reduce pain, specifically pain that originates in the gut.

Many neurotransmitters are produced in the gut. Some neurotransmitters are responsible for the transmission of pain signals, while others help to block pain.

Serotonin is well known as the neurotransmitter being responsible for emotional well-being and a happy mood. A lesser-known function of serotonin is to help block excess pain signals. 95% of serotonin is produced in the gut and one way to increase serotonin production has been found by using probiotics. Lactobacillus helveticus and Bifidobacterium longum can help increase tryptophan which in turn helps to increase your serotonin production.

Endorphins are also well known for helping to reduce pain and the best way to boost endorphins is through exercise. However, the problem for those with endometriosis is that doing any exercise can be really difficult due to weakness, fatigue and pain. This becomes a catch 22 situation. Gentle exercise as we have covered is the best solution like yoga and gentle walking.

Diet, nausea and pain

Quite often certain foods in your diet can trigger nausea and you need to find out which are your particular problem foods. For many women, red meat, sugar and dairy are common triggers for causing nausea and gut distress, as well as causing endo belly – more on this next.

Tips to help with nausea

Many with endometriosis have learnt through trial and error of different remedies that help them manage or reduce their nausea.

These are the most effective nausea remedies:

- peppermint oil capsules
- peppermint tea
- ginger tea
- lemon water
- Zofran
- removing dairy
- removing red meat
- Dramamine - motion sickness med
- Sea Bands/Motion sickness bands

To gain relief from nausea you need to try different remedies until you find what works best for you. Once you start to improve your health by healing your gut and removing your trigger foods, your symptoms of nausea should improve, along with other distressing symptoms of bloating and pain.

Endo Belly/Bloating Help

We now move on to endo belly which causes some very distressing symptoms and is one symptom that is etched into my memory. Endo belly is most notably known to cause really severe swelling and bloating of the abdomen, along with pain and discomfort.

The bloating with endo belly seems to come on in attacks for most, which means there are triggers that set off this distressing symptom. Studies show that as well as constipation and diarrhoea, bloating is the most common GI symptom of the disease.

There are various possible causes why women with endometriosis experience bloating. For instance, endometrial tissue could be near your bowel and this will cause symptoms and distress in that area. If endometriosis infiltrates your bowel, it can cause bloating, constipation, nausea and lots of pain.

Other causes of bloating can include SIBO, Leaky gut, Candida, inflammatory foods, low digestive enzymes, histamine intolerance, excess estrogen and endometriosis adhesions. So, there are many possible reasons for endo belly and something you will need to investigate to get to the cause, and keeping a diary of your symptoms, food intake, supplements used and so on will help to give your clues.

Food and inflammation

As we know, endometriosis causes inflammation which can include having an inflamed gut. The main foods that tend to cause inflammation are sugar, dairy and gluten which can add to the problem. Your gut may also suffer from long-term drug intake with pain-killers and hormone drugs which can upset your delicate gut flora, and an imbalance in your gut flora will mean the functions of your gut will be out of whack.

Also, if you slip up and eat those foods that are your trigger foods, then you will soon know about it – with a nasty attack of endo belly. You really need to learn what your trigger foods are and take note each time you have a flare up. You will soon build up a list of the foods that cause problems for you. If you have been prudent and done the Elimination diet then you should have thoroughly assessed your dietary needs and will know what you are safe to eat and hopefully this means a reduction in your bloating.

Remedies for endo belly

These are some of the self-help measures you can use to help with the inflammation and distress of endo belly.

Probiotics – I mention probiotics often, and as well as helping to heal the gut and balance your gut microbiome, they have been found to help with the bloat and inflammation of endo-belly.

Diet – eating an anti-inflammatory diet and stopping gluten and dairy will help to reduce inflammation and can help reduce endo belly. I get regular feedback from women I work with saying they have a big reduction in their endo flares and bloating after they have changed their diet and left out trigger foods.

Digestive enzymes – these can help to relieve symptoms of pain and gut inflammation with endometriosis. Also, the action of helping you to digest food will take some of the work-load off your digestive system and help you absorb nutrients.

Bromelain - helps you to digest protein and reduces inflammation – comes in supplement form on its own or can be found in a digestive complex.

Serrapeptase - aids in the removal of scar tissue and cysts and can also help reduce inflammation – a topic we have covered earlier.

Water - Water has many benefits and is essential in keeping all of your organs functioning properly. It is amazing how quickly the body can become stressed if you become dehydrated, and having sufficient water will help to keep your digestive system functioning better. Water keeps the food you eat moving along through your intestines and it keeps your intestines smooth and flexible as well.

Peppermint tea – peppermint tea is great. It helps with gut distress and bloating. Many with endometriosis say that peppermint tea also helps relieve cramps with their periods. Peppermint also helps with inflammation and aids with digestion.

Fibre – Balance your intake of fibre between soluble and non-soluble fibre foods - the soluble fibre will help to keep you gut hydrated with fluid, while non-soluble fibre will absorb fluid and slow the transit of waste through your system.

Pycnogenol - Reports of improvement of endo belly symptoms have been noted by some when taking pine bark extract (pycnogenol) taken twice a day. Pycnogenol is the trade name for an extract of French maritime pine bark.

The inflammation-calming effect of pycnogenol has been demonstrated by a decrease in inflammatory markers such as CA-125. A 2007 study printed in the Journal of Reproductive Medicine revealed promising results for the use of Pycnogenol in the treatment of endometriosis.

Castor oil packs – as we have covered earlier, placed on the abdomen, castor oil packs can really help with inflammation and pain and can be very soothing.

These are just a few ideas to help with the pain and distress of endo belly. You may need to experiment to see what works best for you.

Endometriosis & Constipation

While we are covering topics regarding gut issues, the problem of constipation really must be included, especially as this is yet another common symptom that causes much distress.

The issue of dealing with constipation combined with endometriosis is very close to the heart for many sufferers. It is not clear why constipation is so common, but many illnesses and diseases seem to cause this distressing problem, and sometimes constipation can be caused as a side effect of the drug treatment you are using.

The gut seems to take a real hit from endometriosis and there are many causes – inflammation, emotional distress, negative hormones that effect the gut, Candida, drug treatment, laparoscopy bowel prep and digestive sensitivities like gluten – the list just seems to go on and on.

Added to this, there is the pain from inflammation in the general pelvic cavity area, and pain caused by gastro-intestinal infiltration of the disease. When combined with constipation this can lead to a lot of stress as well as pain and discomfort.

Here are some tips that can help

- You need extra fluid in the intestines. Magnesium helps to draw fluid INTO the gut and will help to soften the stools.
- Extra Vitamin C will help as it has a mild laxative effect and taking vitamin C daily will support your immune system.
- When you have a laparoscopy for endometriosis you will be given a bowel prep medication to take before the operation. This usually consists of a powder that cleans the out the gut ... thoroughly!!! This will also strip out the good bacteria. Adding back good bacteria will help rebalance your gut and digestive system.
- Additionally, many women with endometriosis have been prescribed anti-biotics for the early mis-diagnosis of IBS, and taking these drugs will have undermined the health of your gut micro-biome. Taking probiotic supplements will repair the balance and over time will eradicate the bad bacteria.
- Balance your intake of fibre between soluble and non-soluble fibre foods - the soluble fibre will help to keep your gut hydrated with fluid, while non-soluble fibre will absorb fluid and slow the transit of waste through your system
- Use a Squatty Potty or a small foot-stall. When we squat this enables a particular muscle to relax in the pelvis which removes the kink in the lower colon. This makes it much easier for faeces to pass through. I personally use a small foot-stall, and it really does help, and I have feedback from others saying they have had great improvement in combatting their constipation by using a Squatty Potty.

Endometriosis & Insomnia

Suffering insomnia on top of endometriosis just adds insult to injury. When you're desperate to get some rest and you can't sleep really is the last straw. It was something I suffered myself really bad when I had endometriosis and it went on night after night. I often felt really hot with a burning sensation in my solar plexus, which I feel was an imbalance in my hormones. In fact, as well as dealing with pain, having high estrogen can be another cause of insomnia.

I had to use various calming herbs to help me sleep which helped on most nights and allowed me to get some sleep. Interestingly, it was during the full-moon that my insomnia was at its worst as well as when I was pre-menstrual. It was not until my body started to recover and come into balance that my insomnia gradually improved – but I remember the sleepless nights so well.

Often the cause of insomnia with endometriosis is due to suffering pain keeping you awake, but the more we can resolve your pain, the more it will help to combat your insomnia.

Hormones and insomnia

Both high estrogen and low progesterone can be a cause of insomnia.

Many hormones are processed in the liver where specific substances are absorbed into the blood stream and waste is broken down and eliminated. When there is too much estrogen in your body, the liver has to work overtime. This can cause restless sleep.

According to Traditional Chinese Medicine (TCM), the liver is most active at night from 1am to 3am. If you tend to have trouble sleeping during these hours, an overloaded liver (due to high estrogen levels or excess toxins) could be the cause.

As we know, when you have endometriosis it is common to have estrogen dominance, therefore getting your hormones into balance will help towards resolving your sleep issues. Measures you can take to help with insomnia caused by hormone imbalances can include doing a liver detox, improve estrogen metabolism/clearance with supplements like DIM, avoiding xeno-estrogens and improving your progesterone levels with nutrients that support progesterone production.

Other hormones

Insomnia can also be caused by high cortisol, which will definitely keep you awake. Suffering from on-going pain can cause an increase in cortisol levels due to the stress on your body when trying to cope with pain.

There are however many natural remedies and herbs you can try to help calm your system and assist you to get some vital sleep.

Some of the solutions you can try include:
- Calming herbal remedies
- Calming sleepy teas
- Homeopathic remedies
- Relaxing bath with aromatherapy oils and Epsom salts
- CBD oil
- Reduce you use of technology late at night
- Use blue-light blocking glasses in the evening
- Castor oil pack
- Meditation
- Amino acids like tryptophan and gaba
- For racing thoughts try the supplement of theanine

- Melatonin supplement
- Block out all light in your bedroom
- Make sure your bedroom is cool

If one idea or supplement does not work then try something else. If you are stressing out about your situation then try meditating in a calm environment. You will find many guided meditations on YouTube that can help you to relax.

Make sure you follow good sleep hygiene and not use your mobile phone late at night as the blue light from your screen can block your natural melatonin production. Aim to go to bed at the same time every night so that your body gets used to the routine. Also getting up at the same time can help to set your circadian rhythm. Using bright light therapy in the morning not only helps with SAD (seasonal defective disorder) but can help to set your melatonin patterns.

Be patient and try different remedies. If you can start to gain relief from your pain through natural remedies combined with some of the suggestions above you should hopefully start to get your sleep back on track. Improving your sleep will also help improve your immune system.

Herbs & Supplements To Aid Sleep

Here are some of the best herbs and supplements to help insomnia and to aid relaxation

Valerian Root - Studies have found that valerian is one of the best natural solution for insomnia. In addition to insomnia, Valerian can help with anxiety, stress and headaches. Another interesting benefit of Valerian is that it can help to relax the muscles of the uterus, so it can help with sleep as well as help with menstrual cramps.

Passion Flower - In addition to having a calming effect on the central nervous system, passion flower also acts as an anti-spasmodic on the smooth muscles of the body. Passion flower is very effective when used for insomnia and results in a restful, relaxing sleep with no grogginess the next morning.

Lemon Balm - As well as being available as a relaxing tea, Lemon Balm can be used as an herbal supplement to aid sleep. It has a natural relaxing effect on your body and mind, as well as improving cognitive performance.

California Poppy - California Poppy can help provide mental calmness, decrease anxiety and restlessness, and help you get a good night's sleep. It is most often used as a tincture and you can also purchase it as an herbal supplement.

Hops - Most commonly known as a flavouring in beer, Hops have long been used as a remedy for restlessness, nervousness, and sleeplessness, and hops-filled pillows are often used for insomnia.

Wild Lettuce - Often used for insomnia and restlessness, and particularly good for children due to its safety record, Wild Lettuce can be taken as a tincture or as a supplement. Wild Lettuce also has effective pain-relieving benefits.

Essential oils for sleep

Certain essential oils have calming and relaxing properties and can help you unwind to help you drift off to sleep. Try some of the following oils rubbed into your wrists and on the soles of your feet before bed. You can use more than one oil and make yourself a bedtime mix by adding 4/5 drops of each oil into a small bottle of almond carrier oil.

Lavender – can help to slow down your nervous system and decrease your heart rate and blood pressure, which helps you fall into a deep sleep.

Valerian - in addition to helping you fall asleep faster, Valerian essential oil may improve the quality of your sleep, so you wake up feeling more rested. Caution - this oil smells quite bad, so the best place to apply it is the bottom of your feet.

Roman Chamomile - the essential oil of Roman Chamomile has been found to be effective in helping to reduce stress, and can also be used to combat mild cases of insomnia.

Bergamot - this essential oil signals to your system that it is time for bed by slowing your heart rate and lowering your blood pressure. Plus, it reduces anxiety and stress.

Ylang ylang - rubbing a small amount of Ylang yang onto your pressure points can help relieve stress and make you feel less anxious too. This can make it easier to drift off to sleep.

Sandalwood - sandalwood has sedative effects, reducing wakefulness and helps increase the amounts of non-REM sleep

Other issues that can cause insomnia

Sometimes our sleep is thrown out of balance caused by outside influences which can include:

- artificial lighting
- man-made emf
- tech stimulation
- blue light from laptops and phones

There are ways you can rebalance your circadian rhythm which will pay off once you become more strict with yourself and maintain a healthy routine. This can include:

- 20-30-minute walk outside in the morning
- Avoid the use of sunglasses as often as possible
- Open windows, allowing more natural light in
- Use 'f.lux' app on your electronics at night
- Use blue-blocking glasses after sunset
- Use orange/red lightbulbs in evening
- Use candlelight or fire in evening
- Do not use your phone or laptop after 10pm

A Special Mention About Melatonin

We usually think of melatonin as a sleep supplement, as it is the natural substance produced in the brain that increases in the evening to help trigger sleep. However, melatonin is also a powerful natural detoxifier, especially of excess or **harmful forms of estrogen**, and has been researched as a valuable hormone to aid in treating endometriosis. Melatonin also has powerful antioxidant and anti-inflammatory effects in the body.

In one study, melatonin encouraged the shrinkage of abnormal endometrial tissue during melatonin therapy and was able to reduce re-occurrence of endometriosis even after the therapy was discontinued.

In Brazil, researchers studied 40 women with endometriosis by dividing them into two groups. One group were given a placebo and the other group received melatonin supplements over an eight-week period. At the end of the study the results showed a dramatic difference. The women taking melatonin experienced a 40% reduction in pain, improved sleep and 80% less need for other analgesic medications.

In the study, the use of melatonin was able to help with the following:

- Reduce chronic pelvic pain due to endometriosis
- Reduce pelvic pain during menses and during sex
- Reduce pain during urination and with bowel movements
- Led to an overall 80% reduction in the need for pain medication in the women taking melatonin

Women in the melatonin research group also reported substantially improved sleep and a greater sense of wellness on morning waking. What is even more encouraging is that during animal studies, melatonin led to regression and shrinkage of endometriosis tissue.

In summary to the research Dr Tori Hudson says:

'Melatonin is well tolerated by most patients and appears to represent an effective option for pain symptoms related to endometriosis. This study demonstrated that melatonin at 10 mg/day reduces endometriosis associated chronic pelvic pain, including a reduction in pelvic pain, pelvic pain during menses, pain during vaginal penetration, pain during urination and pain during defecation that is statistically and clinically significant.'

With research results as favourable as this, it is worth considering adding melatonin to your natural treatment plan for its multiple benefits – the research has noted that it can help shrink endometriosis tissue, reduce pain and support your sleep at the same time.

How to use melatonin: It is recommended to start at 1-3 mg/day, taken in the evening as it obviously helps aid sleep. For the research program it was suggested to build up to 10 mg over a month, taken at bedtime. At this dose, melatonin supports the body's natural detoxification processes. It is advised to talk to your doctor or natural therapist before using melatonin to ensure there are no contra-indications with any other medication or treatments you are using.

Endometriosis & Fatigue

Fatigue is really common amongst those who suffer endometriosis, and I felt it was one of my worst symptoms. I used to feel as though the life force had been sucked out of me and I could hardly do anything. I found it really distressing and wondered what exactly was wrong with me. It wasn't till I started to recover that my energy began to return. But it really was a life sapping type of fatigue.

But what causes such awful fatigue? In part, it's your body's response to illness. It is a natural response to make you STOP so that your body can focus on dealing with the illness, disease, injury – whatever has caused the problem. If you were to continue as normal your body would not have the energy to put into healing.

Some in the medical community feel that the fatigue with endometriosis is caused primarily by chemical reactions in the body when trying to deal with pain. Personally, I feel it is more complex than that, and the fatigue has more than one cause.

Fatigue itself can cause a range of symptoms some of which you may not consider being caused by your fatigue. This can include muscle and joint pain, headaches, difficulty in concentrating, insomnia, nausea and even heart palpitations.

Apart from the fatigue that is caused by endometriosis and your body trying to deal with the disease, here are some other possible reasons for ongoing weakness and fatigue including:

Low blood sugar and hypoglycaemia, low vitamin D levels, Thyroid problems and hypothyroidism, nutritional deficiencies, adrenal fatigue and low cortisol, anaemia and low iron levels and one issue that is hard to avoid sometimes – poor sleep!

Cytokine release has been noted as another possible cause of fatigue.

'The fatigue women feel is (likely) because of the inflammation caused by the excess endometrial tissue, which sets off a variety of immune responses,' says Karli P. Goldstein, DO, the assistant medical director of the Endometriosis Foundation.

To conclude - there is a strong relation between dealing with illness and disease and feeling very fatigued, as it takes a lot of energy when the body is trying to cope with pain and inflammation. By recovering your health with safe and gentle remedies, your energy will steadily and gradually improve as the stress on your body is reduced.

Thyroid Problems & Endometriosis

Having just looked briefly at some of the possible causes of fatigue associated with endometriosis, let's look at this subject further as thyroid issues can often be overlooked and go undiagnosed.

Maybe some of the symptoms of endometriosis are in actual fact symptoms of a thyroid disorder. The most common thyroid disease among women with endometriosis is hypothyroidism, or underactive thyroid.

Women are at greater risk of developing thyroid problems - seven times more than men. This difference would appear to relate directly to the different hormonal make-up of women. The risk of developing thyroid disease increases with age and for those with a family history of thyroid problems.

What does the thyroid do?

The thyroid is a small butterfly-shaped gland, located in your neck, wrapped around the windpipe, and is located behind and below the Adam's Apple area. The thyroid produces several hormones, of which two are key: triiodothyronine (T3) and thyroxine (T4). The thyroid is the engine of the body and provides the energy in all your cells.

The thyroid does not work in isolation, it is part of a comprehensive hormonal feedback process, which goes like this ….. the hypothalamus in the brain releases something called Thyrotropin-releasing Hormone (TRH). The release of TRH tells the pituitary gland to release something called Thyroid Stimulating Hormone (THS). This THS, circulating in your bloodstream, is what tells the thyroid to make thyroid hormones and release them into your bloodstream.

Once released by the thyroid, the T3 and T4 hormones travel through the bloodstream. The purpose is to help cells convert oxygen and calories into energy. So, when the thyroid is not functioning properly, then insufficient levels of these active hormones are released into the bloodstream, which leads to poor conversion in the cells into energy. This is what causes the lethargy and tiredness associated with hypothyroidism, along with a host other symptom.

What exactly is hypothyroidism?

The most common cause of hypothyroidism is an auto-immune condition which is known as Hashimoto's Thyroiditis, in which antibodies begin to attack the thyroid and gradually make it inactive. There are other causes of hypothyroidism like post-partum hypothyroidism or issues regarding the pituitary gland, but the most common cause is auto-immune Hashimotos's Thyroiditis.

There is much speculation that endometriosis could be an auto-immune disease, and the added development of certain thyroid diseases in women with endometriosis seems to make sense of both conditions developing - as both conditions relate to the immune system, and both relate to a delicate hormonal balancing act.

Symptoms of Hypothyroidism

The symptoms of hypothyroid depend on how severe the imbalance is in the thyroid, your age, your general level of health (enter endometriosis into the equation!), and how hypothyroidism affects you uniquely.

In general, the common symptoms are:

Fatigue, weight gain, low motivation, heat and or cold intolerance, headaches and migraines, dry skin, hair loss, brittle nails, irritability, anxiety, and panic attacks, decreased memory and concentration (poor oxygen levels in the cells), constipation, irritable bowel, low sex drive, insomnia, allergies, slow healing and many more.

Of course, the big problem here is that many of these symptoms are similar to some of the symptoms associated with endometriosis. The best course of action as I said earlier is to get tests to check the levels of hormones being produced by your thyroid.

If your thyroid problem is due to hormonal imbalances and you have low thyroid levels you will need to take thyroid medication to support the function of your thyroid. This can include T4 (thyroxine), T3 (the active thyroid hormone), or Natural Desiccated Thyroid (which contains all the hormones needed to support thyroid function which more closely resembling your natural hormone production).

Most doctors today do not often prescribe the natural thyroid medication and prefer to prescribe synthetic T4 only, which is a precursor hormone that has to be converted into the active hormone of T3, most of which takes place in the liver. If your liver is compromised in any way it can prove difficult to convert the T4 into the hormone your body needs – the T3.

Endometriosis and the Thyroid

In one particular medical survey, **42%** of women with endometriosis had an under-active thyroid gland. This figure is usually 5% in the general population. It also appears that thyroid antibodies are higher in women with endometriosis, which is an indication of hypothyroidism.

Dr. Lee (the pioneer of Natural Progesterone Cream treatments) reasoned that thyroid and estrogen oppose one another. Excess estrogen can cause your food intake to be stored as fat in the body. Thyroid hormone causes fat to be burned as energy. When a woman is estrogen dominant this will encourage further development of fat build-up. This constant opposition between the two hormones could lead to symptoms of hypothyroidism for women with estrogen dominance.

When Dr. Lee treated women with Natural Progesterone Cream for PMS, who also had suspected hypothyroidism, he found that their hypothyroid symptoms disappeared. This success was due to correcting the levels of estrogen by the use of progesterone cream. This implies that too much estrogen in the body interferes with thyroid hormone action.

The significance of this imbalance in hormones (between the thyroid hormone and estrogen) for women with endometriosis, is that if the estrogen dominance is addressed through treatment to increase progesterone (with natural progesterone cream), then many symptoms can be alleviated.

This is especially relevant of the ongoing symptom of constant tiredness, that nearly all women with endometriosis seem to suffer on a daily basis. In essence, it appears that women with endometriosis do not have hypothyroidism - what they are suffering from is probably a disturbance of the activity of their thyroid caused by estrogen dominance.

But you <u>do need</u> to get tested with a full Thyroid blood panel that tests all your thyroid levels, as well as thyroid antibodies to check for auto-immune Hashimotos's Hypothyroidism.

Iron levels and thyroid

There are a few more pieces to the puzzle to make your thyroid work properly. You need to have optimal iron levels for thyroid hormones to get into your cells. Having endometriosis can cause low iron levels due to heavy periods, so a full iron panel blood test is needed at the same time as checking your thyroid.

Cortisol and thyroid

Additionally, your cortisol levels need to be in range. If your cortisol is too high or too low it can affect the function of thyroid hormones. Cortisol increases the active thyroid hormone (T3) and T3 increases cortisol effect - they work in partnership with the cells. It is also known that cortisol and T3 are both required to increase mitochondria energy production, which is another topic regarding fatigue and endometriosis we cover further.

Unfortunately, most doctors do not believe in adrenal fatigue unless you have very high cortisol caused by Cushing's disease or very low cortisol caused by Addison's which can be life threatening.

I have seen numerous adrenal stress tests from clients showing adrenal glands that are on their knees with very low cortisol levels, causing debilitating symptoms of severe fatigue and weakness and sleep disruption.

One important point about adrenal fatigue and symptoms, both high and low cortisol can show with very similar symptoms, so you cannot guess – you need to test otherwise you could be setting yourself up for more problems if you start using any supplements with the incorrect benefits i.e., supplements can be used to lower cortisol and specific nutrients can be used to support cortisol production.

Need for testing

The best and most reliable test is the cortisol saliva test which measures your levels at 4 times over the day to check your body is producing cortisol in a proper circadian pattern.

Your cortisol should be highest as you wake to get you going in the day, and should be nearly at the bottom of the range so that you are able to sleep.

Most doctors will not request a saliva test for cortisol and will only do a blood test. The blood test is not accurate as it measures your total cortisol that is circulating in your blood stream, but this is not measuring the cortisol that is bio-available for your body to use. Whereas the saliva test DOES measure the cortisol that is bio-available, and these tests are even used by NASA due to their accuracy. It is your adrenal glands that produce cortisol, among many other hormones, and the test is usually called the Adrenal Stress test.

The link between your thyroid levels and your cortisol is part of what is called the HPA axis – which is the Hypothalamus / Pituitary / Adrenal Axis. The relationship of the different hormones produced by these glands is very complex and needs to be in balance for everything to function properly.

To get more advice about thyroid disease, cortisol testing and additional information regarding thyroid health there are links to websites for advice at the end of the book. You will find advice where to purchase tests if your doctor will not run the required tests.

Supporting Your Adrenal Glands

Your adrenal glands can take a real knock when you are stressed as we have just covered. They do a lot of work in providing your body with life sustaining cortisol, as well as a host of other hormones including DHEA, testosterone, progesterone, estrogen, pregnenolone and adrenaline.

Cortisol is important for your immune health because it reduces inflammation, it prevents your blood glucose levels from dropping too low, and helps to regulate your blood pressure, as well as providing energy. Additionally, as we have already covered you need optimal cortisol levels for your thyroid hormones to work properly.

As mentioned earlier, you cannot guess the levels of cortisol as both high and low cortisol can produce the same or similar symptoms. However, you can do much to support your adrenal glands with some basic nutrients.

Your adrenal glands store the most vitamin C of all organs in your body. Taking 500mg of Vitamin C daily will provide the support your adrenal glands need. Also, B vitamins, sodium and potassium are needed to support healthy adrenal hormone production.

To make life easier you can make an adrenal cocktail drink to provide the nutrients that will support your adrenal glands, which includes:

- 4oz of orange juice
- 1/4 teaspoon cream of tartar - to provide potassium
- 1/4 teaspoon of fresh ground Himalayan sea salt - to provide sodium as well as additional minerals
- Mix in glass and drink

Alternatively, you can use 8oz of coconut water in place of cream of tartar You can use camu camu powder in place of orange juice if you do not want to use orange juice as camu camu is very high in vitamin C.

Additional support

Another natural support is Nutmeg essential oil and is used by rubbing over the area on your middle back where the adrenal glands are located. Nutmeg is well-known for assisting adrenal gland function. This oil has adrenal cortex-like activity, meaning it supports the adrenals for increased energy. It also helps to balance both the nervous system and the immune system.

Here are some of the findings from data collected from the world's largest research registry on endometriosis.

- Chronic fatigue syndrome is more than 100 times more common in women with endometriosis
- There is a high rate of thyroid disorders in women with endometriosis, as well as their families. Hypothyroidism, which involves an under active thyroid and causes mental and physical slowing, is seven times more common
- Other autoimmune diseases which are seen significantly in women with endometriosis and their families, include Rheumatoid Arthritis, Lupus, Multiple Sclerosis, Meniere's disease
- Fibromyalgia, which is characterised by widespread body pain and tiredness, is twice as common
- Allergic conditions are much higher, occurring in approximately 60% of women with endometriosis

From the finding above is seems obvious that the immune system is playing a major role in all these health issues related to endometriosis.

Chronic Fatigue Syndrome (CFS)

Or is it mitochondria dysfunction?

We now dig deeper and look at another possible cause of fatigue. Very often when suffering endometriosis combined with severe fatigue, it can really feel like you are being hit with Chronic Fatigue Syndrome. Many articles at endometriosis websites discuss the problem of fatigue with some speculating that those with endometriosis may in fact suffer CFS, but could there be another root cause?

Mitochondria and fatigue

Previously we looked at other possible reasons for fatigue like low iron, thyroid issues, or your body simply working hard trying to cope with endometriosis. However, the stress on the body trying to cope with disease can cause other functions to go out of kilter. One such system is the mitochondria function.

Mitochondria produce power throughout your body. Trillions exist throughout the body and as these power producers become less effective or fail, you lose the ability to produce efficient energy and this leads to many health issues. Your mitochondria are responsible for the synthesis of your sex hormones and vital energy producing hormones including your thyroid and cortisol.

> *'Much of the bodies energy - over 90% comes from the mitochondria in cells. As well as energy production, other functions of mitochondria include cell growth, steroid synthesis, and hormone signalling. Mitochondrial dysfunction has been associated with many seemingly unrelated conditions including diabetes, cancer, autoimmune disorders, thyroid problems, liver sluggishness and adrenal fatigue.'* Dr Lam

Damage to your mitochondria can be caused by nutritional imbalances, physical trauma, toxic chemicals, infections and many pharmaceutical drugs including antibiotics, painkillers and antidepressants. Oxidative stress can also cause damage to mitochondria being triggered by inflammatory foods, pesticides, smoking, mould and even Lyme disease. Additionally, to emphasize the issue of everything in the body being inter-related, if the microbiome of your gut is not optimal, you are not absorbing the nutrients you need for mitochondrial function.

Research articles and CFS

There are a number of research articles regarding the link between endometriosis and mitochondria disfunction, looking at various malfunctions in energy systems. The conclusion of one research article, which was based on primate studies found *'Endometrial mitochondrial energy production and metabolism were decreased in endometrium and endometriosis tissue.'*

More research is obviously needed into the link between mitochondria function and endometriosis, as there does seem to be an association between the disease and energy production.

Dr Myhill, a UK doctor who has a special interest in working with CFS patients has written extensively on the subject and feels that mitochondria function is the key to addressing CFS. The typical medical advice is there are no standard tests to diagnose CFS. However, Dr Myhill discusses a specific test, that is not commonly available, called the 'ATP Profile', which can test for mitochondrial function.

The treatment regime she recommends is based on vitamins, minerals, diet, and sleep. She also discusses specific nutrients that are needed to support mitochondrial function which includes D-ribose, CoQ10, acetyl-l-carnitine, NAD, magnesium and B12 injections.

You can read more about her article on CFS and Mitochondria at her website, which I have added here rather than it getting lost in the reference links at the back of the book:

https://www.drmyhill.co.uk/wiki/CFS_-_The_Central_Cause:_Mitochondrial_Failure

She has also written a book on this topic *'Diagnosis and Treatment of Chronic Fatigue Syndrome and Myalgic Encephalitis: It's Mitochondria, Not Hypochondria',* which is available in paperback as well as Kindle.

I am not recommending you rush out and purchase the supplement recommendations, however, some of these supplements can be helpful to take on a daily basis, especially CoQ10 and magnesium. It is interesting to think that part of the problem of fatigue with endometriosis could actually be caused by malfunctions in the mitochondria process and not simply fatigue caused by battling disease.

Mitochondria damage and psycho-active drugs

Mitochondrial damage caused by drugs and toxins is an increasing problem. Many (and I mean many) with endometriosis tend to use a variety of psycho-active drugs to help with anxiety and depression without being aware of the potential long-term damage they can do. There is no shaming here, I just want to make women aware of the harm that these drugs can do to the entire body.

I put my hand up, as I was on Prozac myself for about a year due to depression when I had endometriosis, but I weaned myself off as I did not want to be reliant on chemicals to make me 'feel better'. It was not till a few years later that I learnt of the harm these drugs can do.

These drugs can cause far-reaching damage to your mitochondria function which can produce a multitude of disabling symptoms. These drugs are also responsible for depleting many vital nutrients which compounds the problem of mitochondria damage.

Symptoms Associated with Mitochondrial Dysfunction

Muscles: muscle weakness, cramping, muscle pain, poor muscle tone, vision problems and eye muscle weakness.

Brain: developmental delay, mental retardation, autism, dementia, seizures, anxiety, depression, and other neuropsychiatric disorders

Nerves: neuropathy (burning, pains, pins and needles), acute and chronic inflammatory demyelinating disorders affecting multiple nerves, loss of reflexes, neurologically induced digestive problems like GERD, constipation, and pseudo-bowel obstruction

Gastrointestinal: vomiting, constipation, irritable bowel, trouble swallowing foods or liquids.

Kidneys: loss of protein/amino acids, magnesium, phosphorous, calcium, and other electrolytes, proximal renal tubular dysfunction.

Heart: cardiomyopathy, heart failure, rhythm problems.

Liver: low blood sugar, non-alcoholic fatty liver disease and difficulties with blood sugar regulation, liver failure.

Endocrine: diabetes and exocrine pancreatic failure/pancreatic insufficiency, parathyroid failure, adrenal insufficiency, hyperthyroidism, hypothyroidism

Fatigue: relentless fatigue and weakness. Fatigue is unrelieved by rest. Exercise intolerance may occur.

Drugs that are known to cause mitochondria damage:

Anti-inflammatory and pain medications – aspirin, acetaminophen/Tylenol, diclofenac, fenoprofen, indomethacin, and Naproxen

Anaesthetics and steroids – bupivacaine, lidocaine, and propofol

Antibiotics - Fluoroquinolones (Levaquin, Cipro), tetracycline, minocycline, chloramphenicol, and aminoglycosides

Antidepressants - amitriptyline (Elavil), fluoxetine (Prozac, etc) and citalopram (Cipramil)

Antipsychotics/Mood Stabilizers - Chlorpromazine, fluphenazine, haloperidol, risperidone, quetiapine, clozapine, olanzapine, and lithium

Antianxiety – Alprazolam, Xanax, diazepam, and Valium

From the book; '*Antidepressants, Antipsychotics and Stimulants*',
by Dr. David W. Tanton, Ph.D

Considering the serious damage these drugs can have on your entire system, you are advised to come off these drugs to help recover your health. The longer you stay on these drugs the more damage they will do. Many of these drugs have to be weaned off slowly and carefully with guidance and support of your doctor.

To mitigate the damage, you can support the function of your mitochondria with nutritional support. Once you have discontinued your use of these drugs, doing a detox will help speed your healing and aid recovery from the damage that has been caused.

Coping With Painful Sex

The distressing problem of painful sex with endometriosis is very familiar to many women and sometimes this leads to women avoiding intimacy altogether. The pain suffered during sex is often caused by inflammation or adhesion's in the pelvic cavity. Penetration and other movements related to intercourse can pull and stretch endometrial tissue, particularly if it has grown behind the vagina or lower uterus.

Many women find that certain positions are better than others. For example, when a woman is on top, they can control the depth and speed of penetration, allowing them to determine a comfortable pace.

Here are some tips that may help:

- Make sure you are really fully aroused before penetration as it is less likely to cause pain, because you are properly lubricated.
- Full arousal also causes the vagina to elongate and the cervix to move further up and therefore you are less likely to hurt sensitive areas, such as the Pouch of Douglas or the pelvic organs.
- If you have problems with a dry vagina, try a natural lubricant such as vitamin E oil or Almond oil.
- There are lube products on the market for this purpose, but they do not feel very natural, whereas oils tend to feel nicer. It is quite safe to use these oils; the rule of thumb - never put anything on your body that you would not put inside your body.
- Having penetrative intercourse at certain times of the month. It may be less painful in the week after ovulation, or in the 2 weeks following a period.
- Try different positions for intercourse as this will alter the angle of penetration and in turn will alter the sensation of pressure inside your body to other areas
- Remember, that you do not always have to aim for penetration to enjoy a loving sexual relationship
- Make more special time for love making - have a warm bath together, light some candles, and try to get as relaxed as possible

Keep discussions open with your partner

It is important to discuss the issue of painful sex with your partner. They may not be aware how much pain you are suffering, especially if you are good at concealing your endometriosis pain on a daily basis.

Being open and communicating with your partner is vital to help reduce the emotional impact that can occur when intimate relations suffer. The goal is to foster genuine and open communication, to ensure that sex is pleasurable and free of pain for each partner.

Dealing
With Stress,
Emotions
& Your
Finances

'Healthy living is not just what you eat,
or how much you exercise.
It is also about your mental health.'

Anonymous

Looking After Your Emotional Wellbeing

The mental toll caused by endometriosis is immense and is often unrecognised. The emotions women suffer can include depression, anxiety, panic attacks, suicidal thoughts, low self-esteem, loneliness and avoiding everyday events or situations which could trigger negative thoughts and emotional reactions. These are emotions I am familiar with and have some painful memories of those days.

There is the constant stress on a daily basis of dealing with the symptoms of pain, inflammation, abdominal distress, fatigue and generally feeling really unwell. Going through this day in, day out is enough to cause severe depression.

Add to the daily grind of symptoms is the worry about jobs, finances, medical costs and future financial insecurity. The financial impact can be huge for many sufferers with the constant worry about the ability to be able to keep working. Medical bills can very quickly add up especially when living in a country where there is no free medical care or the treatment you need is not covered by insurance.

There is also the huge stress that can be placed on close personal relationships, which can be seriously affected around problems concerning painful sex and intimate relations. This can often lead to the breakdown of relationships and can end marriages.

All these factors added up can really put severe strain on emotions and will only get worse without some sort of support being provided.

When I had endometriosis, I suffered a myriad of emotional states. I used to suffer distress, depression, anger, bitterness, jealousy, resentment ... you name it .... I felt it. My distress built up to such a fever pitch at one point that I had what can only be described as a minor fit.

I was laid in bed one night and my mind was going round and round and I was very stressed, and suddenly there was a loud BANG inside my head, and the upper part of my body jolted off the bed. It was absolutely terrifying. Luckily my boyfriend was with me at the time to calm me down. But the shock and distress resulted in me crying and crying for over an hour – it was deep, despairing sobbing, with lots of emotional pain and despair being let out. I spoke to my doctor after, and asked what he thought I went through and he felt it was something similar to a mild seizure and this was my brain trying to deal with the stress.

Therefore, I fully understand how deep the emotions can run with this disease, and having support is crucial to help you navigate the deep emotions this disease can cause. So, I don't write this book providing shallow platitudes about healing and recovering your health. Because I have been in the trenches too, and you have to dig deep, get support (and I mean lots of support) and with time you will start to come out the other side.

'You may need to consider getting some help'

Natural therapies for anxiety

There are certain natural therapies that can help manage the emotional aspects of dealing with the stress of illness. Homeopathy is a very good choice and has a huge arsenal of different remedies that can be used for very specific emotional imbalances. A homeopath will take a very detailed description of symptoms, both physical and mental and will then prescribe a remedy, with some of these remedies working at a very deep level. As your symptoms change and improve, then your treatment will also change as layers of healing take place.

Other remedies that may help include acupuncture, which can release emotional blocks and help balance the body. Aromatherapy is very powerful and many essential oils can help with different emotions and calm your central nervous system. Having an aromatherapy massage is very beneficial to help release tension and various oils have a beneficial effect on mood.

One interesting observation - you may also find that your anxiety and depression will reduce when you remove gluten from your diet and start healing your gut. This is due to the intricate connection between the mind and the gut.

Supplements to help anxiety

SAMe - One really beneficial supplement to help with depression is SAMe (S-adenosylmethionine). SAMe is the synthetic form of a compound that is produced naturally in the body from methionine (an essential amino acid) and adenosine triphosphate (an energy-producing compound). SAMe is used to help with depression, fibromyalgia, anxiety and pain – all of which makes this a good supplement for those with endometriosis. Additionally, SAMe can also help to support liver health by helping to increase glutathione.

St. John's wort - Another supplement known to help depression and anxiety is St John's Wort, known to be as effective as antidepressants but without the side effects. It's important to note that St. John's wort is known for interacting with lots of medications. This is especially true for blood thinners, birth control pills, and chemotherapy medications.

Valerian root - This herb is often used in herbal sleeping tablets for its calming and sedative properties, but Valerian also can calm anxiety. Valerian can be used in the day in small doses to calm the nerves or used as a calming tea.

Chamomile - This is another remedy used to help with sleep and anxiety. Recently, a study was conducted comparing chamomile extract with placebo for treatment of generalised anxiety disorder. After 8 weeks results showed that people with anxiety had a significant reduction in their anxiety taking chamomile

Thyme - Thyme is a great source of lithium and tryptophan. Both can help as mood stabilizers and aid sleep. Thyme can be found as an herbal tea or used externally as an essential oil massaged into the body mixed with a carrier oil.

Probiotics - Interestingly certain probiotics can affect mood – it is now commonly known that the gut is the second brain. Supplementing with Bifidobacterium and Lactobacillus strains for 1–2 months can improve anxiety, depression and memory.

Support from others

Finding others in the same situation as yourself can be very empowering and provide great relief to know that you are not alone in this struggle. Joining some of the online forums, message boards, Facebook groups or other social media resources can give you a life-line to provide you with support, share experiences and learn tips that have helped others. Don't go through this alone … you need emotional support.

———————~———————

Counselling To Support Your Emotions

Counselling and therapy should be included as part of your treatment to help you cope and provide emotional support because as we know, this disease really takes its toll on your emotions.

Counselling is also recommended especially as 1 in 4 people with endometriosis have considered suicide, and it has been found from patient surveys that 86% deal with depression and anxiety as a result of having this disease.

Likewise, chronic pain is extremely damaging to people's mental health and the mental impact of illness and pain is just as important as the physical. There is specific help in the form of pain psychology, which is a type of clinical psychology designed for those with chronic pain and injuries and is very different to regular therapy.

It involves the implementation of treatments for chronic pain, which include traditional therapeutic and behavioural techniques like guided imagery or meditation. This approach to therapy helps you to accept your pain as something you can't always control, help you cope mentally and assists with breathing and distraction techniques.

'You need an 'objective' listener'

It is valuable to talk to friends, family, or your partner, but these people have a vested interest; they may not be able to listen objectively and may have the tendency to interrupt you while you are in full flow, which can be quite destructive and deflating for you emotionally.

Also, their own emotions will weigh in on the situation, especially if they have been trying to support you with the emotional burden of this disease.

Therefore, it is the value of having someone who will really listen that is important in counselling. By expressing your needs, worries, your anger, and all your other emotions, you are giving yourself the chance to vocalise and clarify what action to take.

Releasing the burden of endometriosis

Dealing with endometriosis really is a huge burden on the emotions. This burden could prove too much not only for yourself, but also to pour out onto your loved ones. By seeing a counsellor, some of this burden can be lifted.

Counselling may also help you decide what action to take with regard to your treatment and what actions and decisions you need to take in life regarding issues like work, finances and other practical issues.

You need a sympathetic trained counsellor and ideally one who has experience helping those with serious illness. Counselling is not about giving advice or solving your problems. A good counsellor will help you to explore your feeling and emotions and allow you to talk openly and freely.

When choosing a counsellor, you need to ask about training and qualifications, and whether they belong to a professional body. It is essential to trust your counsellor, and that you feel relaxed with them. Otherwise, the process will be counter-productive.

Is This Going To Be Expensive?

Many feel that going the natural route is going to incur lots of added costs - going organic, replacing your toiletries with chemical free options, using natural period products, going to a natural therapist and so on. Let's have a bit of a reality check and look at your options.

Let's break this down:

Going organic - many more food producers are now producing organic foods and this has led to prices becoming more competitive. Considering that certain convenience foods can be expensive, especially if you are buying those ready meals that only provide a meal for one night, then stopping the use of these convenience foods you will be saving money.

Once you get into the cooking habit you can cook in bulk and make ready meals to freeze for another day – this works out cheaper for ingredients and cheaper for your power consumption.

Changing your toiletries - Do you really need those umpteen bottles of face creams and body lotions. As we have covered earlier, you can make your own natural body products using natural ingredients and essential oils. And many oils make great perfume. If you shop around you will find some competitive prices for cosmetics and body products that are much safer, using limited chemicals and often produced with organic ingredients.

Using natural period products - if you changed over to reusable pads, then you are going to actually save money. Once you have made your initial purchase, you do not need to buy any more pads for quite a while. Of course, you could try making your own and there are instructions online how to do this and I have added a link to a website with instructions at the back of the book.

Going to see a natural therapist - the advice and support you gain from seeing any natural therapist goes beyond just supporting your physical health. You will also be given emotional support and sometimes be provided with some insightful advice and guidance.

You may be able to find a natural therapist who is flexible with their payment policy or be able to have treatment at a reduced cost. My own homeopath was well aware of my financial issues and we were able to maintain my healing program by seeing her only every three months.

Another possible option is you may be able to barter or negotiate for your treatment costs. Have you got any particular skills you could exchange for treatment? Maybe you have computer or website skills you could offer in exchange - if you don't ask, you won't know what is possible.

If it is beyond your finances to see a natural therapist, you could gain more insights and advice by reading up on the topic yourself. You will find many introductory books for different natural therapies.

This does not mean you will start self-treating, but you may learn of some helpful and safe home remedies.

If your finances are tight, then when it comes to Birthdays and Christmas, ask your family and friends for gifts that will help your symptoms like a new TENS machine, a healthy food box full of treats or a donation towards some natural therapies.

And finally ....

Let's face it, how many pairs of shoes do you have in your wardrobe that you have never worn, or clothes you have only worn once? We are all guilty of buying stuff we don't need or don't use. But when it comes to your health - *you can't put a price on it.*

A Few Financial Tips .....

Even though we are discussing going the natural route for your endometriosis, you may still need surgery depending how serious your disease has progressed, and this can incur considerable costs, especially if you live in country that does not provide state health care.

Here are a few suggestions ....

Get a clear understanding of your insurance policy

Talk to your company's insurance representative at work if you are still in work. Review your coverage choices and policy benefits. Make sure you understand what your policy covers.

Federal Programs

There are Federal programs that can provide assistance. It can be a lengthy application process, but once you are approved, you can receive coverage that will help. Ask your local health services office about Medicare, Medicaid and Social Security Disability Insurance.

Trust Funds and Grants

Some of the large Trust Funds provide financial assistance for those in need. Most of them have specific criteria, or will only provide for certain diseases or particular circumstances (i.e. funds for Veterans). It is worth doing your research to find what is available. I am unable to provide details of any particular grants and trust funds here, as this requires specific research and can depend where you live and your particular circumstances.

Sliding Fee Scales

Some physicians still actually work with fee scales and payment plans to assist their patients. Ask your doctor about lowering the costs of your office visits and payment plans for visits, test, procedures etc.

A Closer Look At Financial Help

Having just had a quick look at sources of financial help for treatment costs, I want to go into a bit more detail about searching out trust funds and grants for special health issues.

When I had endometriosis, I was desperately strapped for cash and sometimes was living hand to mouth to get by. It was my homeopath who suggested I looked into grants that help those with health issues and having financially difficulties.

I was lucky and was successful in securing a grant for a good quality juicer which meant I could start making my own healthy juices. I later obtained a grant that allowed me to purchase a new bed as my old one was long past it and was not helping with my insomnia.

What type of grants are available?

There are many grants available for individuals, for specific needs and they come from a variety of diverse sources. There are grants for educational needs for those on low incomes, grants for families suffering hardship and grants for the disabled for specific needs. No doubt there will be other grants available.

As endometriosis is a disabling disease, I was able to quantify my own grant application by classing myself disabled. I was actually in receipt of Disability Benefit at the time, which validated my application. However, I feel a letter from your doctor will suffice for some grant applications.

It will totally depend on where you live as to what financial assistance is available. Some Trust funds are very geographically specific, while others are targeted more for certain health issues.

I feel it is well worth pursuing financial assistance from trust funds and grant bodies. Usually, their forms are nowhere near as difficult or lengthy as forms from the statutory bodies. Most trust funds and grant aid organisations will not give you a lump sum to spend on on-going health care costs i.e., 6 months' supply of expensive supplements. What they prefer to fund is larger single items like equipment, wheel chairs, and special adaptations in the home for disabled access.

For example, you could apply for:

- A juice extractor or quality food processor to help you with your diet needs.
- Some Trusts will provide finance for essential household items, and this could include a new bed, washing machine, cooker etc.
- Medical equipment is commonly covered and this could include a TENS machine.
- There are grants for disabled individuals to help them set up home-based businesses, so you could apply for financial help with additional computer equipment to do this.
- There may even be some trusts who will actually finance your on-going medication/supplement needs – do your research and you should find a trust/grant source to help you.

For a lot of women, it is difficult to hold down a job, or you may have difficulty maintain credibility in your job due to the amount of sick-leave you have taken. These issues can be highlighted when you apply to any Trusts funds.

Some of these Trusts have a lot of money and they are there to help people in need, so make use of them. Considering the profits of the top pharmaceutical companies, perhaps you should focus your research to see if any of them have grants for the disabled.

Getting Creative With Your Finances

OK, we all love to buy new clothes, but sometimes this can lead to buying clothes we don't actually wear or spending money we do not have – been there, done that, got the T-shirt!

Have you thought about upcycling all those items in your wardrobe you do not wear? I know this guide is about natural remedies for endometriosis, but the knock-on effects are wide and far reaching, and many with endometriosis end up having financial issues, which is why I have included this topic – it is one issue I am SO familiar with – which bill do you pay first, and how do you prioritise your spending?

Upcycling- reuse what you have already

Upcycling your clothes can be huge fun and brings out your creativity. Pull out all those clothes you do not wear and lay them on the floor. Look to see which fabrics go together; or could you combine that old denim jacket with some lace and make an individual feminine top. If an item doesn't fit cut it up and combine with another piece of clothing to make something new.

Have you simply got bored with a piece of clothing? Add some lace, braids, tassels, embroidery, mix and match buttons round a neck-line – the possibilities are endless, and like I say can be such fun. You can get a lot of ideas online and you may find books on the topic.

Getting creative can extend to making your own jewellery, which is something I love to do. The range of beads available on eBay or Esty is amazing or you can buy old jewellery from charity and thrift shops to recycle.

Be careful though because you can get hooked! But if you get good at this you could start to sell your own creations online. Don't worry if you make mistakes or find your work does not 'float your boat'. It's a learning curve and you simply dismantle what you have made and start again.

I have already mentioned the idea of asking if you can exchange your skills instead of paying for treatment. If you have good creative computer skills and writing skills, you could start to sell your creative services on Fiverr which has become more professional these days, and some people are getting plenty of work.

There are also plenty of opportunities to work from home using your computer, which gives you the chance to work at your own pace, and to manage any flare days. Ask other members at endo support groups of the online/work at home jobs they do and they can provide you with advice, contacts and websites with more information.

You may be aware of some of these ideas already, but sometimes we forget what we already know, if you know what I mean. Anyway, I digress. The bottom line is that there are many creative ways you can try to manage your financial needs.

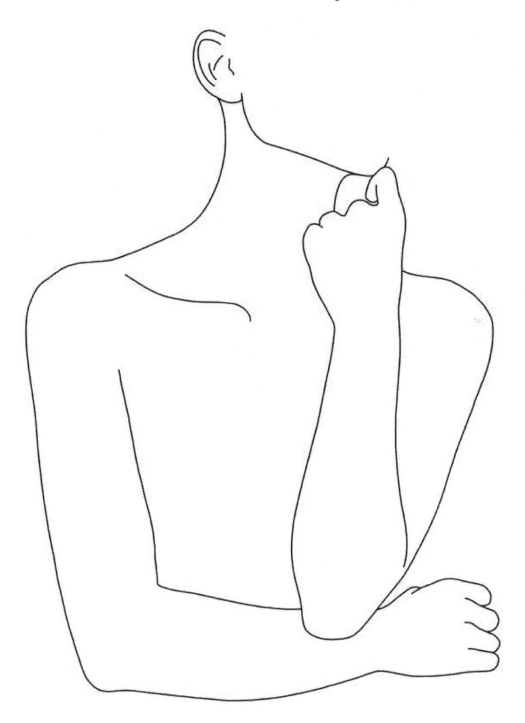

What's In Your Survival Kit?

When trying to manage illness, we all need to have certain resources and tools to help us get through, and those with endometriosis have learnt to have certain tools readily on hand.

Here are a few suggestions

- **Books, books and more books** – endometriosis books, diet and nutrition books, recipe books, natural healing books, positive reading books
- **Heating pad or hot water bottle** – to help with your pain, and you will also need a hot water bottle when doing castor oil packs.
- **TENS machine** – really helpful for muscle pain, menstrual pain and they are also really helpful for back pain
- **Message boards and support groups** – make sure to ask questions and get involved, even if only for emotional support. Some of these groups have a wealth of information.
- **Big bag of Epsom Salts** – soaking in the tub with Epsom salts at night will help with muscle pain and calm you for sleep
- **Essential oil kit** – we have covered the many uses of aromatherapy to help endometriosis – this includes pain relief, insomnia, skin preparations
- **Pain relief teas** – peppermint tea is really helpful for bloating and ginger tea can help with nausea
- **Loose clothing** – to help when you have endo belly and nothing seems to fit
- **Supplements** – a selection of specific supplements to help your symptoms. Introduce any supplements gradually and give them a chance to work as they are not a quick fix like pharma meds
- **Keeping a diary** – to track your symptoms and really helpful to monitor any changes and take note of any modifications you have made in your treatment. The more symptoms you track, the more insights you will gain.
- **Castor oil pack kit** – very helpful to calm your pain and inflammation and also helpful to detox your liver. Ideally used before bedtime as castor oil packs can be calming
- **Calming herbal teas** – use at night to help aid sleep, or use in the day when feeling stressed
- **A Netflix account** – so you can binge watch TV when you are having a flare
- **Support** – try to maintain contact with friends, especially those who have not left you high and dry because you are no longer able to socialise like you used to. Get your family on-board and get them educated about this disease so they understand what you are going through.
- **Your doctor** – you can't do this all alone and you need to have your health monitored by your doctor. Explain to your doctor that you are trying more natural things to help your

endometriosis – your doctor may be understanding, as some are now supportive of using natural treatments to manage health problems.

What About Surgery?

Despite my focus on going the natural route, I am not opposed to surgery when needed. Surgery is necessary to obtain an accurate diagnosis, and will be needed to remove the disease and hopefully stop it developing further.

However, you can do a lot to improve your health with safe natural alternatives and life-style changes, but if your endometriosis has reached such a level, then surgery may be needed to remove the cysts, adhesions and endometrial implants.

What does concern me is that many women have surgery to remove endometriosis and it often returns sometime later. Many women are having multiple surgeries – this is a common situation. For this reason, it is desirable to try and manage this disease more naturally, and to stop the ongoing cycle of repeated surgeries or using toxic drug treatment with their many side-effects.

'Surgeons can cut out everything except cause' Herbert Shelton

Which type of surgery is best?

The consensus now is that excision surgery is the best surgical treatment for endometriosis, however there are long waiting lists to see an expert excision surgeon, and there are only an estimated 300 specialists worldwide. Even with the best excision surgery, the disease can still return.

Excision involves cutting out endometrial lesions until the surgeon reaches healthy tissue. Unfortunately, most gynaecological surgeons are not qualified to perform excision as most are not educated correctly in the distribution and appearance of the disease.

The other common form of surgery for endometriosis is ablation, which burns the tissue using heat or lasers, but this type of surgery has disadvantages as it does not allow the surgeon to see where disease tissue ends and often only the surface tissue is removed. This can leave deeper diseased tissue untreated.

Research has assessed the different outcomes between ablation and excision surgery, and they found that excision surgery led to more improvements than ablation for patients in the following 12 months after surgery.

However, according to endometriosis.net many women experience a recurrence of endometriosis by 5 years after surgery (20-40%, according to some studies). This is why it is important to aim to calm the disease through natural remedies and reduce your need for more surgeries.

If you are looking to have surgery, ideally you need to find an endometriosis specialist who has experience in excision surgery, and you will find details of endometriosis specialists in the resources section.

A quick note about supplements before surgery

You are advised not to take any supplements for two weeks before surgery, especially those that are blood thinners. This includes serrapeptase, turmeric, omega 3 oil, vitamin E, gingko biloba, as well as certain spices including ginger, garlic, cayenne pepper.

What if you can't have excision surgery?

Sometimes excision surgery is not always an option. Either because of money constraints, your location or not being able to find an excision surgeon. Some women have opted for ablation surgery and have found relief, while others have used a recommended surgeon from the *Nook list of excision specialists and have had a bad experience.

Also, some women have opted for a hysterectomy and it has been successful for them, whereas many have gone down the path of having a hysterectomy only to find the disease returns. It needs to be noted that having a hysterectomy should only be considered for adenomyosis, and hysterectomy is not a treatment for endometriosis.

This is why endometriosis is so difficult to manage, difficult to treat and difficult to know which is the best treatment option to use for the best outcomes.

You can only do what is manageable for you, and by implementing the self-help measures we have covered here, you can take more control of you own health and with patience you will see results.

And don't let your surgeon or GP 'talk down to you', as they often do, thinking you know little about your disease. LET THEM KNOW that you know plenty about endometriosis – you are living it day in, day out. Talk to your surgeon candidly and ask LOTS of questions about their experience and the antic-ipated outcomes of surgery, and how to manage your health and recovery after surgery.

And finally, an interesting observation about surgery – it has been discovered that if your surgeon and the medical team talk positively about your surgery while the operation is taking place, it has been found that patients have a better recovery and can actually heal quicker. Once again, your subcon-scious is listening in. So, ask your medical team to talk kindly!!

*Nook surgeons are endometriosis surgery specialists listed at Nancy's Nook – which is a Facebook page offering information and advice about recommended endometriosis surgeons.

'Expert excision of Endo implants removes disease, but lack of disease does not equal good health. Diet, lifestyle, mindset and integrative therapies need to be addressed in the treatment plan to get the best possible outcomes.'

Dr. Andrew Cook MD

Laporoscopy Surgery Advice

Having just covered the topic of surgery for endometriosis, I felt it would be helpful to include this guide to help you prepare for laparoscopy, including tips to help speed your recovery. This advice can be found on the website, but I felt it would be useful to include it here for your reference.

If you are going into hospital for the first time to have a Laparoscopy for endometriosis, it can be a worrying time. The emotional anxiety about what the surgeon may find will cause as much concern as the actual process of having surgery.

Preparation

If you are well prepared the whole experience will be less traumatic and frightening. It is also vital to obtain information from your consultant or gynaecologist as to what they intend to achieve during your laparoscopy. If you are unclear of anything they say, ask for a better explanation. You will no doubt have many questions and concerns. Write these down and discuss them in your pre-op appointment with your consultant.

You will want to know what surgical options there are for the treatment of endometriosis. This will depend on the training and experience of your particular consultant. You will also want to know how your consultant can deal with different stages of the disease. Each laparoscopy will be different as no two women are the same, and there are no set patterns to this disease.

Prepare Practicalities

There are many small but very useful things you can do to make the whole process of undergoing surgery and recovery much easier. Much of this is about preparing practicalities around the home and your life so that you can focus on resting and recovery when you get back home.

- Prepare your food stocks so that you have all the provisions you will need. If you live with a partner then they will be doing the cooking, but if you live alone you need to buy in some frozen or instant meals. Better still, cook and freeze your own meals in advance.
- Clean your home the day before surgery, then you come home to a nice environment
- Change the linen on your bed the day before surgery, again for the pleasure of nice clean sheets, and you will not be capable of changing the linen for at least a week by yourself
- Make sure you have a supply of sanitary towels, pain killers, hot water bottle, ensure your Netfix subscription is up to date as you will be binge watching TV.
- Make sure you have 2 or 3 loose fitting outfits. You will not want to be wearing anything tight, especially round the abdomen
- Start taking extra Vitamin C for about 2 weeks prior to the operation - this will help your body deal with the anaesthetic as well as help with healing
- Purchase Homeopathic Remedies - Arnica 30c - you will use this to assist healing and relieve pain after surgery. Phosphorus 6c - to relieve vomiting after anaesthetic
- Purchase some throat lozenges - to help with the sore throat caused by the tube which is put down your throat during the operation
- Inform friends and family of your operation date and the time you expect to be back home. This will allow them the opportunity to keep in touch and see how you are. Also put your phone by the bed for easy reach.
- Obviously if you have children you will have to make child care arrangements. If you have pets, especially a dog, you need to make arrangements for dog walking

Prepare Yourself

- The day before - eat light and healthy and drink lots of fluids. Do not eat or drink anything after 12.00 midnight the night before surgery
- Do not smoke or chew gum after 12.00 midnight If your surgery is scheduled for later in the day, it is advised to have some supper around 11.00pm so you are not totally starving throughout the next day
- Your doctor or consultant will probably ask you to do an enema in the evening to clean out your bowel. If more severe endometriosis is suspected, then a full bowel prep may be required. You will be given instructions on this during your pre-op office visit. Preparing the bowel with a purging agent such as Magnesium Citrate is often followed by an oral antibiotic and enemas. While unpleasant, this procedure minimises the risk of surgical complications from bowel injury during surgery.
- Pack a hospital bag including: warm, loose clothing to wear after the operation, wash-kit, sanitary towels, something to read if you have to wait around for your turn in theatre, clean socks to keep your feet warm during surgery. Leave your wallet and valuables at home.
- Remove all nail polish, remove jewellery and contact lenses

- Ensure that you have a lift home from hospital. If this has been pre-arranged with a friend some time beforehand, ring them a few days before to ensure they remember.
- Take a long warm bath the night before, drink some camomile tea to aid restful sleep, and get a good night's sleep

The Day of Surgery

- Try to get up early, take a shower if you wish and put on comfortable clothing. Do not bother doing much to your hair; it will only be put into a protective cap for the operation. Do not forget that you are not allowed breakfast. Do not wear any make-up, perfume, hair spray or deodorant.
- Arrive at the hospital at the designated time to register. There will be forms to fill in and consent forms to sign. Ensure that you specify what you do NOT want to have done during surgery.
- The process of signing in to hospital on the day of your treatment will vary for different countries, but the actual medical procedure will be similar. You will probably be shown to your bed and given instructions by a member of the ward staff. This usually involves instructions for getting undressed and changed into hospital gowns, putting any belongings into safe keeping, and then advised to wait for consultations with the medical staff. You will get a visit from your consultant and one from the anaesthesiologist.
- You need to discuss with the anaesthesiologist any fears or worries you have. They will ask you about any allergies you may have or whether there is any family history of bad reaction to anaesthesia.
- You will be given a pre-op injection or sedative drug which makes you feel very drowsy and floaty. This helps to alleviate some of the nervousness. This is usually given about an hour before the operation.
- You will arrive at the theatre suite, in a prep room just outside of theatre. The anaesthesiologist will make sure you are ready and will then insert an IV (intra-venous) needle into the back of your hand. A tube is then fitted to the IV ready for the anaesthetic to flow directly into your system. The anaesthesiologist will ask you to start counting backwards from 100, keeping your eyes open. You will feel a cold rush into the back of your hand as the anaesthetic starts to flow into your system. Most people do not get much further than counting down to about 80.

Surgical Recovery

You will not remember anything else until after your operation. Depending on which country you live in, you will either come round from the surgery in the recovery room or you will back on the ward in your bed.

You will be feeling very groggy and unsure of where you are at first. You will then begin to focus your thoughts for a while and will realise that you are back safe in the real world again. You will drift in and out of sleep for a few hours whilst the anaesthetic wears off. A nurse should come and take your temperature and check your pulse and blood pressure at regular intervals.

As you begin to come round a bit more you will start to feel the different pains in your body. You will have pain where the incisions were made; your abdomen will feel sore and painful from the operation as well as being distended by the gas.

The worst pain noted by most women is a sharp stabbing pain in the shoulder. This is a side-effect of the gas that is used to distend the abdomen, which seems to travel around the system. The pain can feel as though a sword has been driven through you. So watch out for this one – it's one thing I remember most about my post-surgery experience.

You need to ask for pain killers if you suffering a lot. You can also be given something to help with the nausea. You need to try sipping some water if you feel up to it. Many people feel too nauseous to let anything pass their lips.

This is a good time to take some Phosphorus - the Homeopathic remedy - to help you stop feeling so queasy. Take one dose every half hour until you start to feel more settled. You can then start to get some fluid into your system and drink some water. You can also start taking some Arnica - the other Homeopathic remedy - to help speed up recovery and reduce the pain.

You will find yourself continuing to drift in and out of sleep very easily for a few more hours. Do try to get up at some point and go to the toilet to urinate. This will sting because of the catheter that is inserted for the operation. If you are having treatment on a day-care basis you will not be allowed to go home until you have urinated. This is to ensure that your system is working correctly.

If you staying at the hospital overnight then you will be given something very light to eat before the day is over. This will help to level out your blood-sugar levels and will improve how you feel.

Your first night will be rather uncomfortable with abdominal pain, feeling groggy from the operation, and an awful shifting pain in your shoulders, which hurts every time you move around. The pain is at its worst when you try to sit up. Do your best to lie still for your first night, and try not to get to distressed about the results of your surgery.

You may have been given your results on the day of the operation but in most cases your consultant will inform you of the outcome the following day if you are staying overnight.

If you are a day-case, you can go home once you feel ready for the journey and the medical staff are happy with your vital signs. Those who are staying over-night will be checked over in the morning and will probably go home around mid-morning.

For your journey home, ensure someone is going to collect you. You will NOT be able to drive yourself. It is a good idea to have a small cushion to hold against your abdomen. This helps to protect you from sudden bumps in the road. It is also advisable and more comfortable to recline your seat slightly.

Get out of the car carefully AND GO TO BED.

Recovery at Home

For the first few days you need to stay in bed and get as much sleep as possible. You will have bleeding which will be similar to having a period, which is normal.

- The incision near the navel can be rather sore. If you have had another incision lower on the abdomen this will also need protecting. Do not wear any clothing that is going to rub on these incisions. Follow your doctor's instructions on cleaning and dressing the incisions and watch for signs of infection.
- The stitches used in the incisions are usually the type that dissolve so you do not need to return to hospital to have them removed
- It can take a few days for the shoulder pains caused by the gas to finally stop. It will also make you belch a lot.
- Your abdomen will be bloated for a few days, but will gradually go down
- The amount of surgical pain and cramping you have will depend how extensive your surgery was. Use painkillers and a hot water bottle or heating pad.
- Just take things steady for the first few days. Try to get up and walk around the house a little bit. You may feel dizzy and weak, but it is better than lying in bed and not moving at all, which will make you feel worse when you do try to get up.
- Your diet needs to be very light and simple for the first few days. You may find that you are constipated which is caused by a combination of the anaesthetic, lack of bodily movement, lack of food intake, and the effects of painkillers.
- Drink lots of fluids, especially pure water, fruit juices, herb teas. Increase your bulk intake after 2 days. It is best not to eat too much at first. Digestion taxes the system and requires energy to take place. It is best to reserve this energy for healing and let your body get over the shock.
- Gradually get back into normal routine over a period of about a week, increasing what you do every day.
- Do not try to bend over to pick things up - it hurts far too much. Bend at the knees instead and drop your weight down to pick things up.
- Continue taking a few doses of Arnica each day to help speed your recovery

Returning to Daily Life

Your healing will be steady and gradual over the period of about 2 weeks before you start to feel somewhat normal again. I would not personally advise going back to work for a least a week, and this is only if you do a desk job. If you do any physical work - which most women with endometriosis cannot anyway - you need to consider having at least 3 weeks off work.

Get Support & Get Involved

Getting support is vital when you have Endometriosis. There are so many social media groups, endo blogs, forums, websites — the amount of advice now is astounding.

It's a good idea to get involved with these valuable resources. Joining forums and support groups will allow you to get much needed advice and feedback, tips about treatment, advice about natural remedies, as well as much needed support.

Many with endometriosis start their own support groups on Facebook, or set up advice pages at Instagram. Writing about your experience with endometriosis and starting a blog can be very thera-peutic, or you could write guest posts for one of the many endometriosis websites.

'Support is so important to stop you feeling so alone or isolated'

You also need support closer to home. You will probably need help with shopping or cooking when you feel bad and have a flare. Don't be afraid to ask. Try to keep your friends 'in the loop'. Unfortunately, sometimes friends can disappear, but if you try to get them educated about this disease, then maybe they will start to understand and can give you more support.

Don't forget to treat yourself sometimes .....

If you have the finances consider giving yourself a treat once in a while. Go for a lovely aromatherapy massage or go for a spa day. If you can't afford it, then improvise at home and have a pamper day— a deep hot bath with essential oils followed by a manicure, and then some healthy snacks and Netflix!

Your Support Team - Let's Look At The Details

To reserve your energies for your healing journey you need to build a support team. Your personal circumstances will weigh-in here as to who will be included on your support team. It will depend on whether you are married or single, working or still studying and other personal situations.

The first and most obvious member of your support team is your doctor, as well as other professionals, for example a natural health therapist, nutritionist, acupuncturist etc. If your doctor is not under-standing of your decision to use the support of natural remedies than maybe you need to look for a more sympathetic doctor.

If you are currently working you will need support and understanding from colleagues and from your boss. Make sure you educate them on the severity of this disease and that it is not 'just a bad period'.

You need to inform them of your circumstances and ensure they know you are not avoiding your duties when you are having a rough patch. See if you can delegate some of your work-load, as and when it is necessary.

If you have lost your job due to taking too much sick-leave, or you have decided to stop working as you could not manage any more, then read the section again about alternative ways of managing finances. There are now many ways to earn money using the internet and many online jobs are available, which may help you get through till you recover your health. The last thing you need now is stress caused by financial difficulties. As I mentioned earlier, other endo sufferers on social media can give you advice where you can find online working opportunities and there seem to be plenty of options.

On the home front, you will need support from your spouse or parents to help you manage when you are not feeling well and unable to do too many house-hold tasks. To ensure you are feeding yourself well, it is good idea to do batch cooking and have some frozen meals ready for the days you do not feel able to cook.

Ask family members to help with grocery shopping, or if you live alone, thanks to the internet, you can now get home deliveries. Also ask your family if they can help with some of the more physical house-hold chores so that you can conserve your energies for healing.

The final part of your support team are your friends. Unfortunately, many friends can disappear into the woodwork when you are dealing with health issues. This seems to be part of human nature and not being able to cope with misfortunes, or not being able to deal with ill-health.

However, if you do have supportive friends that have stuck around, then make sure you keep in touch with them and let them know you appreciate their friendship. Put time aside to be with your friends, as emotional support is very valuable and helpful for the healing process.

To recap – your support network will include: medical professionals, work colleagues, family and friends. If your support network seems thin on the ground due to personal circumstances, like living alone, or most of your friends have deserted you, then make sure you get in touch with the many online advice and support groups. See if there are any support groups near you that meet up, where you will be able to get much needed emotional support.

Timescale of going the natural route

Going more natural to manage endometriosis could take many months for you to start seeing improvements in your health; this depends how far the disease has progressed in your own case. The longer you have been ill, the longer it will take to see improvements. But the options of not striving for recovery do not bare thinking about; more surgeries, more toxic drugs, more expense, more pain, recurrence of the disease, more stress, more heart-ache.

The time span to start seeing success in your healing may seem rather long, especially for those who are desperate for a quick fix. It can take a long time for your body to become diseased, so it will take months to start getting any recovery and reduce the symptoms of this disease. Please think of this time as an investment in the rest of your life.

Do Not Give Up On The Natural Route

Sometimes people can be really impatient when it comes to their health and they want a quick fix. This is understandable, but you need to practise patience and be realistic. I just want to recap the sequence of events of my own healing journey to emphasise my positive message.

To summarise my endo journey ....

- I was diagnosed with severe endometriosis after having a laparoscopy.
- None of the endometriosis was removed during this surgery.
- I was offered hormone drug treatment, to try and calm the disease – which I refused after discovering the potential side-effects.
- At this point I researched in earnest what the disease was, what had gone wrong, what causes the disease, and all the other questions any woman will ask after being diagnosed.
- I then decided to follow a natural route – this included seeing a homeopath every few months, using natural remedies, and being very mindful about my diet.
- I sustained this regime for nearly two years at which point I felt fit, healthy and on top form, except for one niggling 'feeling' that there was just one more 'block' to remove.
- I had a further laparoscopy and the day after surgery my surgeon came to see me and told me I had one cyst on my ovary, which he removed, but that 'all other signs of the disease had dried up' – his words.
- That was the end of any 'treatment' I had for endometriosis, and it never returned.
- My point is that endometriosis can go into remission/be healed, whatever you want to call it. And remember, I had severe endometriosis.

Another piece of the puzzle was my utmost belief and commitment that I *would* get rid of this disease. I stayed focussed on my belief and even if my belief wavered due to a flare up of symptoms, or my emotions faltered, I stuck with it.

I felt I had no option .... Because what was the alternative? You know the answer to that one.

NOT A QUICK FIX .....

I have occasionally been contacted by women who have tried different alternative therapies and have felt let down. They have only felt limited benefit from the therapy they have chosen.

They have not given the therapy a good chance to take effect which requires a suitable time-frame. They may have tried a regime of homeopathy or herbalism or whatever, for a few months and then given up because they were not seeing significant improvements.

People are so used to the idea of a quick fix for things in life, especially with modern medicine. We are all so impatient. But if your body has taken years to become diseased then it will take a while to repair the damage and get your body back into equilibrium and balance.

When it comes to treating and healing diseases modern medicine tends to go in with a sledge hammer, and sometimes does more harm than good. There are the dangers of side effects, some of which are permanent and very damaging to the body (look up the lawsuit cases for patients who have been prescribed Lupron).

Your body chemistry is very delicate and the most delicate chemical system is the hormone system. We all know that endometriosis is fed and activated by hormones. In the human body, it takes only micro-scopic amounts of any given hormone to have a powerful and cascading effect in the body.

These hormones are very potent, and yet the very treatment being offered for endometriosis by modern medicine is synthetic hormonal drugs, which will obviously throw the body into disarray and upset a finely tuned orchestra of natural chemicals in the body.

Please be kind to your body. Healing yourself is simply a matter of being committed. A total commitment to change the way you are doing things. Do not leave it up to others; take control of your own health.

'Healing your body is like peeling an onion – it's about uncovering the layers of ill-health and getting to the root cause'

Let's Recap Some Self-Help Measures

- Maybe start by re-reading this guide again and taking notes. I may have only touched on certain topics that seem significant to you, so you can research these subjects in more detail for yourself.
- Link up with others in forums and social media and make use of these groups and ask questions to get advice and feedback of what has helped them. Be aware that we are all different, and what may work for someone else may not work for you – but you can at least get some recommendations i.e., product recommendations, feedback on surgeons etc.
- Consider having certain tests done, especially if your fatigue or symptoms are severe and you feel something else is 'off'. Tests to consider are thyroid, iron levels and a check for any nutritional deficiencies.
- Change your diet so that you eat an anti-inflammatory nutrient rich diet – preferably starting with an elimination diet to assess your gut health and food triggers.
- A gentle detox is a good starting point for your overall health and will help to off-load toxins in your system. Make sure you are supporting your detox pathways – i.e., supporting your liver, having Epsom salts baths (refer to the detox section).
- Start doing castor oil packs a couple of nights per week – this is a very beneficial and cheap natural remedy which will help with detox and calm inflammation and pain.
- Change you period products to natural options, or you could make your own reusable pads.
- Aim to get support from one or more of the natural therapies, and ensure you choose a therapy where you feel comfortable about the treatment being offered.
- Help your body with targeting supplements that are most relevant to your symptoms, but add them in one by one so you can monitor any benefits.
- Stop using toxic chemicals and change your cosmetics to more natural options, and use less chemicals in your home.
- Start to keep a diary and include treatments started, diet changes, supplements you have tried - this is so important. Also log you cycle, pain levels and any other noticeable symptoms or changes.

A Few More Healing Stories

These stories are included to give you hope and motivation that you too can obtain relief and start to heal your body, and this just a small selection of the stories that have been sent to me over the years.

This first story is a guest article from Stacy Kelly which is featured at the website at endo-resolved, who was finally able to free herself of endometriosis after changing her diet.

Stacy's story ....

'I suffered from endometriosis from the age of 15 until the age of 36. I found out I had the condition after having a large mass on my ovary. I sincerely thought I had ovarian cancer and the fright of that was not something I can explain. It turned out that the endometriosis had formed a cyst on my ovary.

This was discovered at the age of 28 and I only knew about it after I had major surgery. I was diagnosed after surgery and as you see it took many years, during those painful years I lived on painkillers to get by and cope with life as a young woman.

I learned to live in fear of this condition and dreaded every month that would come. After diagnosis, I still didn't understand how to care for this condition, it was after my 8 weeks check-up that I was given a contraceptive to try. I was so happy to be given something that may be of some help to me.

It was a great help actually, I managed to have a life, be normal, and have a social life. The pills however after a while gave me severe side-effects such as suicidal thoughts and deep depression. I should say that this was after changing many brands because each brand had its own side-effect such as migraines, change of my emotional stability.

They had stopped working for me and so I came off them in 2016 after 7 years of taking them. The endo had started creating havoc in my body after I came off the pills, it spread into my anus, it affected my digestive system. I had developed gluten and wheat intolerance and suffered for about 5 years before realising I needed to change my diet.

Once I changed my diet, I realised how much I needed to do that. The pain in my anus went away, my cluster headaches left me and my endo pains eased off. I couldn't explain it but I was happy. I can say right now that changing my diet helped to heal my body, I stopped eating sugary foods, gluten & wheat, stopped having dairy (although I only had small amounts sometimes) but after cutting these things out my life became better.

I mainly adopt a vegetarian diet and live on grains, nuts, seeds etc, I occasionally have chicken or other meats and fish. My endo tummy went away, and I was no longer embarrassed about how bloated I looked.

Endometriosis can be a debilitating condition, please get checked for your painful period and then seek a natural way to treat this condition. Life after endometriosis is great, I do not have to fear if

I am away from home and I have an unexpected period because I do not have those severe pains anymore.'

Success with herbalism

'After 13 years of having to take anti-inflammatory medications for my menstrual cycle, I was not able to function without them. After a ruptured ovary, surgery and extreme endometriosis, my options for a "normal" life involved taking the pill along with an experimental drug that would tell the body it was in menopause or pregnancy, or I could have a hysterectomy.

I used a herbal formula from my herbalist regularly for six weeks. I was two weeks late with my menstrual cycle, so I figured that the formulas were not working either. To my surprise, when I did have my period, I didn't have to use any anti-inflammatory medication. I experienced only one day of cramps that were about 1/10th of the severity that they normally were. Furthermore, I didn't become as sick with nausea or diarrhoea as I usually do. I have been suffering with this problem for many years while thinking that it was never going to go away unless I had a hyster-ectomy. Certainly, at only age 26, that procedure held its own complications and repercussions!

I am very grateful for the opportunity to try an alternative approach that really works! Thank you for my life back!' Monica

Acupuncture and pain control

'Valerie is a 35-year-old single woman. She began to have unusual menstrual pain about five years ago when she was riding a bicycle while she had her period. Recently, her menstrual pain became severe, spreading to the vagina, anus, hips, and inner side of the thigh. A "sinking" sensation in the anus, with abdominal pain and back soreness accompanied the menstrual pain. Often, the pain was severe enough to trigger bouts of nausea and vomiting, and she became desperate for relief.

She went to her regular doctor, who referred her to a gynaecologist. The pelvic examination, magnetic resonance imaging and laparoscopy confirmed that she had endometriosis. The gynae-cologist suggested a hysterectomy, but she refused. She asked for other options. The doctor told her that "acupuncture is effective to relieve pain. Why don't you try it?" She came to my clinic. After three month's treatment with acupuncture and Chinese herbal medicine, her endometriosis was under control.'

. If only I knew that such a non-invasive and totally safe procedure would work so well.'

Acupuncture success

'I seemed to have had painful periods for a long as I can remember. I would be in so much pain that I knew something was wrong. I was also feeling generally unwell. I went to my doctor on and off for about 10 months, until finally I was referred to a gynaecologist. I had a Laparoscopy in the winter of 2017 and I was diagnosed with moderate to severe endometriosis. I had never heard of it before this. I was offered hormone drug treatment and was unhappy about using it.

I had tried using the BCP to regulate my periods a few years before and the hormones really upset my system and I felt really ill. I decided to try acupuncture for the pain as I had read that acupuncture is good for treating pain for lots of illnesses. After 3 treatments I started to feel better. My acupuncturist said we could go further with the treatment with the purpose of boosting my immune system and hopefully to treat the endometriosis. I had regular treatments over the next 18 months and my health gradually improved as well as reducing the pain of my periods. I now have normal periods and last year I gave birth to a beautiful baby boy. I would recommend any woman to try acupuncture if they have endometriosis. I thank my acupuncturist so much.'

Success with Naturopathy

'I asked the doctors what I should do, and they had no answer for me but to give me pain medication, which led to codeine, but eventually nothing could stop the pain. Incidentally, the only time I had a break from endometriosis was when I thankfully got pregnant with my daughter but that was after four miscarriages. After I gave birth to my daughter, the endometriosis came back in two months now worse than ever before.

Finally, I found a naturopathic doctor, who along with her husband runs one of three naturopathic schools in the United States. I started using herbs and in one year had no more pain and am still pain free. Because of the herbs I used, I never had to have surgery, which was the next step - a hysterectomy.

My heart goes out to anyone who suffers with this. You are absolutely correct when you write how the constant pain robs you of a normal happy life. When a person has that much pain, they are miserable and irritable, such a terrible thing to endure. There had been times that I sincerely wanted to die.' Candy

A diet success story from Janine

'I have tried many different treatments to help with my endometriosis, but none of them have been of any long-lasting help. I was diagnosed with a laparoscopy 4 years ago and the doctor removed some of the implants and a few of the adhesions while operating. (I had symptoms of pain for at least 2 years before this).

I was then given hormone drug treatment to put me into a menopause. This helped for a while but the side effects were dreadful. In fact, they seemed worse than my original endometriosis symptoms. I suffered severe weight gain, my skin became very greasy, I had severe trouble with sleeping, and felt really ill most of the time.

I came off the drug treatment as not only did I not want to continue, but I did not want the long-lasting side effects like bone loss. At one time I tried the BCP but again the side effects were awful. I would wake up every morning feeling really nauseous and it would last nearly all day. I tried that for 6 days and gave up.

I did not know what to do to try and deal with this disease. So I decided to give the diet a go as I had read about it on various endometriosis boards and many of the women were saying how helpful it was. I started the diet about 5 months ago and I have never felt better. The pain I suffered for most of the time has almost gone. My pain levels with my period is about 3, on a scale of 10. I feel much healthier and suffer less bloating.

I wish I had tried the diet earlier, but I was under the illusion that medical treatment was the answer. I am now thinking of going to see a naturopath in my area and see if I can improve things even more. I really want to save - or improve - my fertility as I am still hoping and praying to have a family one day.

Girls, do give the diet a try. It is natural, safe and for me has been much better than using the dreadful drugs for treatment with all the awful side effects.'

Where Do I Start?

You can't do this all at once. Just like you cannot totally change your diet in one go. It is easier to make small changes gradually. If you were to go gung-ho and make lots of changes all at once you will not know what is helping and what is not.

Taking small and steady steps will help to ease you into a new health regime. Taking more charge of your own health is really empowering and helps you to feel like you have more control. Starting with diet changes is a very good place to begin, especially as so many others with endometriosis have really good success once they changed their diet (myself included).

Then build from there with steady gradual changes. Ideally you need to start tracking your symptoms from the start as this will give you a benchmark of all the symptoms you have been dealing with.

Write down what changes you want to make and the self-help measures you are going to try. Sometimes writing things down helps to galvanise our thoughts, and the very process of writing your ideas down is a start to making changes. *Don't we all love to make lists!!!*

Write a shopping list for the new food items you are going to buy. Do some online research and check-out where you are going to buy some gentle natural toiletries. Ask at the online endometriosis message boards and support groups of products they can recommend – all these small things are a start in the right direction.

If you take on too much at once or try to make too many changes you may feel overwhelmed – just do this in manageable stages - then you are less likely to give up. If you have any questions feel free to contact me at the website and I will do my best to provide whatever support I can.

The more that you believe that something is going to happen; the more likely it will happen. This is the same with your health. The more you believe that you will recover, the more chance you have of this actually happening.

It is now time to embark on your own journey towards recovering your health. The Chinese proverb says 'The journey of a thousand miles begins with one small step.' Take this journey one step at a time, do not look back, keep your heart and mind fixed on your objective, and you will arrive at your desired destination.

With healing thoughts, Carolyn

Resources

Footnote

Helpful Links

More Reading

References

Footnote

Putting this book in context - endo-resolved was one of the first websites to offer advice about nutrition and natural remedies to help manage endometriosis, and I still continue to learn to this day. It has been very rewarding to offer support to women, helping them to recover their health going the natural route. Putting this book together is now a natural extension of that support, which I hope has achieved its objective.

Endometriosis is a whole-body disease, and this theory is now gaining momentum. Once upon a time this disease was just seen as a gynaecological problem. This disease affects the entire body, therefore, the whole body – physically, mentally and emotionally needs to be taken into account when working to heal the body.

About the advice here

My aim has been to keep this book upbeat and positive. I am all too aware that there are many distressing stories to be found about the day-to-day life of living with endometriosis, but that is not the focus of this book. This book is about providing solutions and hope.

It is not possible for me to advise you which specific remedies or treatments to use, as we are all different, and your particular health issues will be very individual. As we have covered earlier, you may be suffering with additional health problems and these will need addressing.

Additionally, what may work for you may not work for someone else. It is recommended that you seek advice from a natural therapist or nutritionist to help guide you and ensure you are covering all your health needs, even if it is only to get an initial assessment of your health status. From there you will have a treatment plan that is specific for you.

It can be really helpful and supportive to do further reading on natural therapies, nutrition and self-help and there are a few book suggestions a little further on. If you are considering trying any herbal remedies it is advised to get advice from a qualified herbalist or Naturopath, as some of these herbs can be very potent, and any current medication you are taking will need to be checked for any contra-indications.

When working with any natural therapist, always aim to work in partnership with your doctor so that they are kept in the loop and know which treatments you are following. If your doctor is not sympathetic of your decision to use natural remedies in combination with any allopathic treatment then maybe you need to consider finding a more sympathetic doctor. Your health is a priority, and you need people to be on your side.

The content of the book

I included the many feedback stories of successes using natural therapies and diet to provide you with motivation, and help increase your belief of your own possibility of recovering your health. It was one of the things that really helped me during my own healing journey.

The account of my own story of recovery from endometriosis, though it is brief, I felt was sufficient to give you a basic outline to my healing process. I did not want to write up a lengthy account of my story, which could have filled a third of the book. I wanted this book to focus on being an information resource, and one you could dip into for guidance and information.

The advice here may seem to rely on many lists about supplements and treatment ideas, often being repeated in the book. This method of providing advice helps you to find advice that relates to specific symptoms, rather than the other way round.

Heads up - I just want to give a quick note about the spelling in the book, as some of you may find the spelling of certain words different from what you are accustomed to, as this book is written in European English rather than American English – just to clear up any concerns about my literacy skills!

In closing, this book could easily have been much longer as there is so much information that could have been included about natural therapies, gut health, nutrition and healing. I hope I have touched on sufficient topics to cover most bases, and you can now go on to do further research yourself.

What I really hope this guide offers you is a huge dose of confidence and inspiration to using gentle natural remedies, so that you can start to manage this disease more naturally and regain your health. You deserve it.

with love

Carolyn

Lastly, if you have found this book helpful please consider leaving a review where you purchased the book which will help to spread the message about going the natural route. *Many thanks*

Helpful Links

Endo-resolved links:

Website: https://www.endo-resolved.com

Endometriosis Coaching: https://www.endo-resolved.com/endometriosis-coaching.html

Facebook group: www.facebook.com/groups/endometriosisdietandnaturalsupport/

Instagram: https://www.instagram.com/endoresolved/

Pinterest: https://www.pinterest.co.uk/endoresolved/

Other Helpful Links

Nancy's Nook Facebook Group

To find advice about endometriosis specialists

https://www.facebook.com/groups/41813699157461

Finding a functional medicine doctor globally

https://www.ifm.org/find-a-practitioner/

Stop the Thyroid Madness

A good resource for all things thyroid

https://stopthethyroidmadness.com

Links and special offers for tests in USA for thyroid, cortisol and hormones

https://stopthethyroidmadness.com/recommended-labwork/

Tests for cortisol, thyroid and additional lab work for UK – Medichecks

https://medichecks.com

Tests for cortisol, thyroid and additional lab work for UK – Genova Diagnostics

https://www.gdx.net/uk/

Testing for SIBO UK

https://smartsibotest.com

Testing for SIBO USA

https://sibotest.com/pages/index

Comprehensive list of SIBO testing laboratories for USA, UK, Australia

https://www.siboinfo.com/testing.html

Step by step SIBO treatment plan

https://sibosos.com/sibo-recovery-roadmap/

British Homeopathic Association

https://www.britishhomeopathic.org

American Institute of Homeopathy

https://homeopathyusa.org

American Association of Naturopathic Physicians

https://aanmc.org/national-associations/

British Naturopathic Association

https://www.the-bna.co.uk

American Association of Acupuncturists

https://www.asacu.org

British Acupuncture Council

https://www.acupuncture.org.uk

For advice about Low Dose Naltrexone

https://www.ldnresearchtrust.org

Natural period products USA

https://periodaisle.com

Natural period products UK

https://www.earthwisegirlsuk.co.uk

Organic cotton period products USA

https://cora.life

Additional Reading

Endometriosis Books:

'Endometriosis: A Key to Healing Through Nutrition' - Dian Shepperson Mills

'Stop Endometriosis and Pelvic Pain' - Andrew S Cook and Robert Franklin

'The Endometriosis Health and Diet Program' - Dr Andrew Cook and Danielle Cook

'Period Repair Manual' - Lara Briden

'WomanCode' - Alisa Vitti for advice about eating foods in tune with your cycle

Diet and Nutrition Books:

'Recipes and Diet Advice for Endometriosis' - Carolyn Levett

'Vegetarian Cooking Without' - Barbara Cousins

'The Body Ecology Diet: Recovering Your Health and Rebuilding your Immunity' - Donna Gates

Natural Healing and Emotional support books:

'The Healing Power of Essential Oils: Soothe Inflammation, Boost Mood,

Prevent Autoimmunity and Feel Great in Every Way' - Eric Zeilinkski

'Pain Relief without Drugs - A Self Help Guide for Chronic Pain and Trauma' - Jan Sandler

'Quantum Healing' - Deepak Chopra

'Perfect Health' - Deepak Chopra

'The Healing Path' - Marc Barasch

'You Can Heal Your Life' - Louise Hay

'The Road Less Travelled' - M Scott Peck

'Anatomy of the Spirit - The Seven Stages of Power and Healing' - Caroline Myss

'Hands of Light: A Guide to Healing through the Human Energy Field' - Barbara Ann Brennan

References

https://en.wikipedia.org/wiki/Endometriosis

https://www.mayoclinic.org/diseases-conditions/endometriosis/diagnosis-treatment/drc-20354661

https://www.nichd.nih.gov/health/topics/endometri/conditioninfo/treatment

http://endometriosis.org/treatments/

https://www.verywellhealth.com/natural-treatments-for-endometriosis-89275

https://endometriosisnews.com/2017/08/10/5-natural-treatment-options-endometriosis/

https://www.ncbi.nlm.nih.gov/pubmed/15254009 - red meat and endometriosis link

https://www.ncbi.nlm.nih.gov/pmc/articles/PMC3626048/ - dairy consumption and endometriosis

https://www.ncbi.nlm.nih.gov/pubmed/23334113 - endometriosis and gluten link

https://academic.oup.com/humrep/article/25/6/1528/2915756 - dietary fat and endometriosis

https://www.ncbi.nlm.nih.gov/pmc/articles/PMC6066416/

https://www.medicalnewstoday.com/articles/321471#diet

https://www.medicalnewstoday.com/articles/320630.php

https://en.wikipedia.org/wiki/Phytoestrogen

https://en.wikipedia.org/wiki/Prostaglandin

https://endometriosis.org/news/research/prostaglandins-cox2/

https://www.ncbi.nlm.nih.gov/pmc/articles/PMC6501744/

https://www.health.harvard.edu/staying-healthy/foods-that-fight-inflammation

https://pubmed.ncbi.nlm.nih.gov/23334113/

https://pubmed.ncbi.nlm.nih.gov/30383387/?from_term=naturopathy+and+endometriosis&from_pos=1

https://pubmed.ncbi.nlm.nih.gov/29077705/?from_term=acupuncture+and+endometriosis&from_pos=1

https://pubmed.ncbi.nlm.nih.gov/29944729/?from_term=acupuncture+and+endometriosis&from_pos=2

https://www.ncbi.nlm.nih.gov/pmc/articles/PMC5017946/

https://www.verywellhealth.com/natural-treatments-for-endometriosis-89275

https://www.ncbi.nlm.nih.gov/pmc/articles/PMC3950373/

https://pubmed.ncbi.nlm.nih.gov/30383387/?from_term=naturopathy+and+endometriosis&from_pos=1

https://pubmed.ncbi.nlm.nih.gov/31335707/?from_term=chinese+medicine+and+endometriosis&from_pos=3

https://pubmed.ncbi.nlm.nih.gov/29077705/?from_term=acupuncture+and+endometriosis&from_pos=1

https://pubmed.ncbi.nlm.nih.gov/29944729/?from_term=acupuncture+and+endometriosis&from_pos=2

https://www.ncbi.nlm.nih.gov/pubmed/15254009 - red meat and endometriosis link

https://endometriosisnews.com/2018/06/26/higher-endometriosis-risk-linked-red-meat-study/

https://www.ncbi.nlm.nih.gov/pmc/articles/PMC3626048/ - dairy consumption and endometriosis

https://www.ncbi.nlm.nih.gov/pubmed/23334113 - endometriosis and gluten link

https://academic.oup.com/humrep/article/25/6/1528/2915756 - dietary fat and endometriosis

https://www.ncbi.nlm.nih.gov/pmc/articles/PMC6066416/

https://www.medicalnewstoday.com/articles/321471#diet

https://www.ncbi.nlm.nih.gov/pubmed/29734542

https://integrativewomenshealthinstitute.com/will-drinking-aloe-juice-help-my-digestion/

https://natural-fertility-info.com/essential-oils-and-aromatherapy-for-endometriosis.html

https://endometriosisnews.com/2017/06/13/8150/

https://www.medicalnewstoday.com/articles/326108.php

https://academic.oup.com/humupd/article/25/4/486/5518352

https://www.ncbi.nlm.nih.gov/pubmed/3110710

https://www.ncbi.nlm.nih.gov/pubmed/11476764

https://endometriosisnews.com/endometriosis-and-immune-system-dysfunction/

https://endometriosisnews.com/2018/01/29/for-endometriosis-pain-relief-try-using-castor-oil-packs/

https://advancednaturopathic.com/news-events/health-articles/benefits-of-castor-oil-packs/

https://www.endometriosis-uk.org/causes-endometriosis

https://www.mayoclinic.org/diseases-conditions/endometriosis/symptoms-causes/syc-20354656

https://en.wikipedia.org/wiki/Prostaglandin

https://www.ncbi.nlm.nih.gov/pubmed/20511671

https://www.ncbi.nlm.nih.gov/pubmed/22003899

https://endometriosis.org/news/research/prostaglandins-cox2/

https://www.yourhormones.info/hormones/prostaglandins/

https://www.medicalnewstoday.com/articles/320630.php

https://en.wikipedia.org/wiki/Phytoestrogen

https://www.ncbi.nlm.nih.gov/pmc/articles/PMC3074428/

https://integrativewomenshealthinstitute.com/gluten-and-endometriosis/

Marziali M, Capozzolo T. (2015) Role of gluten-free diet in the management of chronic pelvic pain of deep infiltrating endometriosis. J Minim Invasive Gynecol

Marziali M, Venza M, Lazzaro S, Lazzaro A, Micossi C, Stolfi VM. (2012) Gluten-free diet: a new strategy for management of painful endometriosis related symptoms? Minerva Chir

https://www.ncbi.nlm.nih.gov/pubmed/23334113 - endometriosis and gluten study

https://www.fertilitytesting.co.uk/use-of-green-tea-as-treatment-for-endometriosis.html

https://clinicaltrials.gov/ct2/show/NCT02832271

https://www.urmc.rochester.edu/encyclopedia/content.aspx?contenttypeid=19&contentid=GreenTeaExtract

Interview with Dr. Phil Boyle, Director of the NaPro Fertility Care Clinic in Dublin, Ireland. (2016). Retrieved from https://www.ldnscience.org/resources/interviews/interview-phil-boyle

https://clinicaltrials.gov/ct2/show/NCT03970330

https://pennstate.pure.elsevier.com/en/projects/endometriosis-a-novel-approach-to-symptom-management-with-low-dos

https://www.ldnscience.org/patients/clinical-trials-in-progress

https://www.cemcor.ubc.ca/ask/endometriosis-and-natural-progesterone

https://www.everydayhealth.com/endometriosis/treatment/progesterone-endometriosis-natural/

https://www.ncbi.nlm.nih.gov/pmc/articles/PMC5077092/

https://en.wikipedia.org/wiki/Prostaglandin

https://www.ncbi.nlm.nih.gov/pubmed/20511671

https://endometriosis.org/news/research/prostaglandins-cox2/

https://www.yourhormones.info/hormones/prostaglandins/

https://www.ncbi.nlm.nih.gov/pubmed/6366808

https://www.ncbi.nlm.nih.gov/pubmed/2647603

https://www.ncbi.nlm.nih.gov/pmc/articles/PMC5790697/

https://www.sciencedirect.com/topics/agricultural-and-biological-sciences/phytic-acid

https://www.mercola.com/article/soy/avoid_soy.htm

http://americannutritionassociation.org/newsletter/downside-soybean-consumption-0

https://www.ncbi.nlm.nih.gov/pubmed/30412246.

https://www.liebertpub.com/doi/full/10.1089/jmf.2018.0160.

https://healthfully.com/63529-herbs-lower-estrogen-levels.html

https://www.livestrong.com/article/324522-supplements-to-reduce-estrogen/

https://www.researchgate.net/publication/237120489_Nutritional_Influences_on_Estrogen_Metabolism

https://www.endonews.com/vitamin-d-and-endometriosis

https://endometriosisnews.com/2016/11/11/ovarian-endometriosis-linked-to-vitamin-d-blood-levels-in-study

https://www.ncbi.nlm.nih.gov/pmc/articles/PMC5189720/

https://www.ncbi.nlm.nih.gov/pmc/articles/PMC6122064/

https://pubmed.ncbi.nlm.nih.gov/31863346/

https://en.wikipedia.org/wiki/Xenoestrogen

https://www.ncbi.nlm.nih.gov/pubmed/21747346

https://womeninbalance.org/2012/10/26/xenoestrogens-what-are-they-how-to-avoid-them/

http://jphs.iautmu.ac.ir/article_523793.html

https://pubmed.ncbi.nlm.nih.gov/30412733/

https://pubmed.ncbi.nlm.nih.gov/23536571/

https://endometriosisnews.com/2019/03/12/resveratrol-helps-reduce-two-enzymes-endometriosis-trial/

https://www.endonews.com/resveratrol-and-endometriosis

https://pubmed.ncbi.nlm.nih.gov/23091400/

https://www.researchgate.net/publication/257958490_Lack_of_evidence_that_essential_oils_affect_puberty

https://roberttisserand.com/2010/04/is-clary-sage-oil-estrogenic/

https://www.researchgate.net/publication/221700049_Changes_in_the_volume_and_histology_of_endometriosis_foci_in_rats_treated_with_copaiba_oil_Copaiferalangsdorffii

https://www.science.gov/topicpages/c/copaiba+oils+obtained.html

https://pubmed.ncbi.nlm.nih.gov/23842934/

https://www.ncbi.nlm.nih.gov/pmc/articles/PMC6330594/

https://www.ncbi.nlm.nih.gov/pmc/articles/PMC6066416/

https://endometriosis.net/clinical/ablation-excision/

https://www.mayoclinic.org/diseases-conditions/endometriosis/diagnosis-treatment/drc-20354661

https://my.clevelandclinic.org/health/diseases/4551-endometriosis-recurrence--surgical-management

https://pubmed.ncbi.nlm.nih.gov/29870739/

https://academic.oup.com/humrep/article/19/8/1755/2356458

https://www.ncbi.nlm.nih.gov/pmc/articles/PMC3374872/

https://www.rbmojournal.com/article/S1472-6483(13)00007-2/fulltext

https://journals.lww.com/md-journal/Fulltext/2020/05290/Effect_of_melatonin_for_the_management_of.60.aspx

https://www.endonews.com/roles-of-melatonin-in-endometriosis

https://www.sciencedirect.com/science/article/abs/pii/S030439591300081X

https://pubmed.ncbi.nlm.nih.gov/29734542/

https://www.medicalnewstoday.com/mnt/releases/137015#1

https://pubmed.ncbi.nlm.nih.gov/1651678/

https://pubmed.ncbi.nlm.nih.gov/17660705/

https://academic.oup.com/ajcn/article/79/3/516/4690160

https://academic.oup.com/humrep/article/22/10/2693/600313

Index

Made in United States
Troutdale, OR
12/11/2024

26246178R00166